RITUALS &
IN NURSING

RITUALS & MYTHS
IN NURSING
A SOCIAL HISTORY

CLAIRE LAURENT

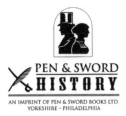

PEN & SWORD
HISTORY

AN IMPRINT OF PEN & SWORD BOOKS LTD.
YORKSHIRE – PHILADELPHIA

First published in Great Britain in 2019 by
PEN AND SWORD HISTORY
An imprint of
Pen & Sword Books Ltd
Yorkshire – Philadelphia

ISBN 978 1 47389 661 1

A CIP catalogue record for this book is available from the British Library.

Typeset in Times New Roman 11.5/14 by
Aura Technology and Software Services, India
Printed and bound in the UK by TJ International

Pen & Sword Books Limited incorporates the imprints of Atlas, Archaeology,
Aviation, Discovery, Family History, Fiction, History, Maritime, Military, Military
Classics, Politics, Select, Transport, True Crime, Air World, Frontline Publishing,
Leo Cooper, Remember When, Seaforth Publishing, The Praetorian Press,
Wharncliffe Local History, Wharncliffe Transport, Wharncliffe True Crime and
White Owl.

For a complete list of Pen & Sword titles please contact
PEN & SWORD BOOKS LIMITED
47 Church Street, Barnsley, South Yorkshire, S70 2AS, England
E-mail: enquiries@pen-and-sword.co.uk
Website: www.pen-and-sword.co.uk

Or
PEN AND SWORD BOOKS
1950 Lawrence Rd, Havertown, PA 19083, USA
E-mail: Uspen-and-sword@casematepublishers.com
Website: www.penandswordbooks.com

Contents

List of Illustrations

1. Nurse from Glasgow Royal Infirmary 1967. (The Herald and Times Group)
2. Nurses' dining room Western Infirmary Glasgow 1960s. (Copyright NHS Greater Glasgow and Clyde Archives)
3. Setting up a blood transfusion; Western Infirmary, Glasgow 1960s. (Copyright NHS Greater Glasgow and Clyde Archives)
4. Student nurses in lecture 1960s Western Infirmary, Glasgow. (Copyright NHS Greater Glasgow and Clyde Archives)
5. Patient being nursed in an iron lung. (Wellcome collection)
6. Student nurse St Helier Hospital, Carshalton, 1943. (Wellcome collection)
7. Inserting a chest drain. (Wellcome collection)
8. West Midlands Sanatoria. (Wellcome collection)
9. Patient in traction. (Wellcome collection)
10. Nurses on a ward early twentieth century. (Wellcome collection)
11. London Hospital badge. (RCN Archives 2015)
12. Royal Infirmary Edinburgh School of Nursing. (RCN Archives 2015)
13. Manchester Royal Infirmary badge 1973. (RCN Archives 2015)
14. Glasgow Royal Infirmary badge.
15. Sam Gamgee who in 1880 invented Gamgee tissue, an absorbent cotton wool and gauze surgical dressing.
16. E3 ward Hope Hospital, Salford 1927. Alice Clegg first on left. (Courtesy of Rosalind Gooley)
17. Headscarf embroidered with the initials of nurses who wore it when they were operated on by surgeon Mr James Sherren at the London Hospital. (Copyright Barts Health NHS Trust Archives and Museum)
18. Nurse No. 1 Ethel Gordon Fenwick. (Courtesy Barts Health NHS Trust Archives and Museum)
19. All kinds of medicines and mixtures made it onto the drug trolley circa 1920s. (Copyright Barts Health NHS Trust Archives and Museum)

Acknowledgements

This book exists thanks to the generosity of all those nurses, past and present, who have entrusted their stories, their memories and best of all their humour to a project that can only be summed up in the question: Egg white and oxygen, why?

Special mention goes to Mary Anne Laurent without whose prodigious memory and endless support this book would not have been written. To my aunt Molly whose reminiscences enlightened me about both nursing and the richness of my own medical/nursing family and to Mary Stiff, my first interviewee, who gave so generously of her time and who has sadly now passed away. Molly and Mary both lent me their nursing text books which proved an invaluable source of nursing rituals.

I would like to thank St Bartholomew's Hospital Set 16 for their contributions, especially Anne-Marie, Jackie, Jacqui, Judy, Liz and Susie. I would like to extend my thanks to The League of St Bartholomew's Nurses, and in particular for the support of past president Professor Maggie Nicol, and to the many nurses from Bart's wider family for their fantastic support, in particular Alison and Alison, Caroline and Caroline, Eileen, Eunice, Gill, Jean, Lee, Paula, Rosie and Thelma. My thanks also to Alison, Berni, Cate, David, Diana, Dianne, Erica, Gay, Gail, Jeanne, Kathy, Kayte, Linda, Liz, Martin, Mary, Melissa, Michael, and Sarah as well as David Barton, Tom Bolger, Natalie Doyle, Christine Hancock and Ann Keen, who shared their memories. You can continue to follow the progress of this book at Facebook.com/Rituals and Myths in Nursing.

Grateful thanks are also extended to:

Wendy Moore and Janet Snell, who provided so much good advice and editorial guidance. To Hina Pandya who introduced me to the dark arts of social media and to Alan who long advocated that I write about nursing and patiently proof-read pages of hospital jargon. To Emma, Victoria and Jake for their support and encouragement.

Archivists, Kate Jarman, Barts Health NHS Trust, Alistair Tough of the NHS Greater Glasgow and Clyde Archives and Louise Williams at Lothian Health Services Archives, for their interest, time and support.

The Royal College of Nursing Foundation, Teresa Doherty, Royal College of Nursing Joint Archives and Information Services Manager. Fiona Bourne, RCN Archives Operational manager and Neasa Roughan, RCN archives specialist.

Disclaimer

For clarity and consistency, the pronoun 'she' has been used when referring to nurses, except when a man is specifically quoted. The pronoun 'he' has been used when referring to doctors and patients except where the gender is specifically noted. It could be said that this sums up the culture still embedded in our hospitals and wider society.

Those who have been quoted have given permission to use their names. In some cases pseudonyms have been used. The names of any patients have been changed to protect their identities.

Preface

Most aspects of basic nursing, including the nurse's approach to the patient are steeped in tradition and passed on from one generation of nurse to another. Too often they are routine without rhyme or reason. They are learned by imitation and taught with little if any reference to the underlying sciences.

Virginia Henderson, 1967

Introduction

Nurses are depicted as female and caricatured as angelic, sexy or fierce. From the tabloids' 'angels' to the *Carry On* films' formidable Hattie Jacques matron and buxom Barbara Windsor, to Nurse Ratched in *One Flew Over the Cuckoo's Nest*, nurses are rarely just people doing a job. They are angels, dragons or sex objects.

This, despite Florence Nightingale leading the charge more than 100 years ago, to establish nurses as a workforce of demure, clean and educated girls, far away from the 'Sairey Gamp' slatternly image of Charles Dickens fame.

While Florence's philosophy of nursing was about building a professional body of educated women with the right personal qualities, it could be argued that Ethel Gordon Fenwick (née Gordon Manson) took the profession to the next level. At the age of 24 in 1881, she became matron of St Bartholomew's Hospital. She formalised the nurses' training and improved their working conditions. She resigned her post in 1887 when she married Dr Bedford Fenwick but campaigned for the next thirty years to establish a nationally recognised register of nurses.

Although it seemed they wanted the same thing for nursing, Ethel and Florence were on opposite sides of the debate about the register. Florence felt it would undermine her philosophy of nursing as being about the right personal qualities and aptitudes. Ethel wanted a more formalised and universal three-year training programme, a more standardised curriculum and a final examination.

In some ways they both won. Formalised training and a nursing register were established in 1919. Mrs Gordon Fenwick was the first name on the register and is known as Nurse Number One and for Florence's part, people still talk today about the importance of vocation in nursing.

The battle about nurse training continues, often dichotomised into education versus compassion as if the two cannot happen together.

Introduction

Nurses themselves are divided on whether their profession should be degree-based as it is now, or an apprenticeship as it was for the best part of 100 years. All are agreed it should be evidence based, as argued by Virginia Henderson.

Nursing grew from a military model of rules to support the actions of doctors and as a result developed a rich culture of rituals and routine – from ward rounds to drug rounds, from preoperative theatre preparation to the cleaning and storing of equipment, from bedmaking to blanket baths. New rituals are developing all the time around technology, the completion of paperwork and the ticking of boxes as recording and checking takes over from doing.

The mention of rituals brings out two sharply divided nursing camps: those who think any sort of ritual implies unthinking behaviour resulting in ridiculous and, on occasion, even dangerous actions, and those who think ritual often has a role to play, offering security and comfort that can be part of the healing process.

This book uncovers both kinds, sharing nurses' stories as they convey how they perpetuated these familiar myths and customs, exploring how they came about, and how they are steeped in the history of health, the military or religion.

I trained in a large teaching hospital in the 1980s and after a long break completed a 'return to practice' course and worked part time in a local district general hospital. My experience is limited to general hospital nursing and therefore so is this book, although I recognise that mental health and community nursing have their own rituals and myths ripe for the telling. I have not included stories from the two world wars mainly because these are so brilliantly covered in other books on the history of nursing, and because coping during the war years brought a whole different brand of rituals and resourcefulness.

Chapter 1

Without Rhyme or Reason

'Wet behind the ears.'

The air was putrid with the smell of urine. It was dark. Even with the lights on it felt heavy and enclosed. At 4 o'clock every afternoon, the cry would go up: 'I need to get home to make my husband's tea,' and, as one, half-a-dozen of the ladies on the elderly care ward at St Matthew's Hospital, Hackney, would make for the door, coats and hats on, empty handbags over their arms. The permanent nursing staff, wise to this routine, would have locked the ward doors just minutes before to prevent a mass exodus of confused old ladies. We students were both bemused and saddened as the ladies clamoured for the life they once had.

Originally a workhouse built in the 1800s, St Matthew's was converted to a hospital about 100 years later, at one time housing nearly 1,000 patients. By the time I arrived in 1981 there were about 180 beds or so, all for elderly patients with dementia – often referred to as 'psychogeriatrics', or psychiatry of old age.

I was a middle-class 19-year-old nursing student previously protected from the fact that people may grow old and poor and have nowhere better to end their days than a dark, smelly hospital ward cared for by strangers. At the time, their care was probably considered quite progressive, but to me it felt as if the old people were being warehoused and I wondered how they felt, how their families felt at having to leave them there and, most importantly, how I would get through the next three months.

All the patients on the ward had dementia and we students had little knowledge of how to care for anything other than their physical needs. For once, we were allowed to chat to them and listen to their stories. Nurses were usually meant to be too busy to talk, but on this kind of ward there was little else to do. At least here there never seemed to be sweeping consultant ward-rounds, or the need to polish the bedpans in the sluice.

Rosie worked on one of the men's wards at St Matthew's. She used to sit and listen to one chap's war stories and when he offered her a Brazil nut from the bag on his locker, she happily took one. It was only when his daughter arrived carrying a box of Callard & Bowser Chocolate Brazil nuts that Rosie began to feel uneasy and slightly queasy. The daughter glanced at Rosie: 'You've not been eating those, nurse?' Rosie said she had. The daughter said: 'Oh Dad, I've told you not to suck the chocolate off the nuts – it's a nasty habit.'

Worse is Kayte's account of one old lady who loved to prank the medical students. She spent hours rolling poo into Malteser size balls and putting them in a Malteser box. The nursing staff had to warn the students not to take one if she offered them.

The physical care of the ladies on my ward at St Matthew's mostly involved encouraging them to wash and to dress in their usual clothes rather than staying in hospital-issue nighties. This was quite a battle, and once a week, they were all 'persuaded' to have a sit-down shower. This usually involved a lot of kicking and screaming from our charges. Once in the shower, at least three nurses were required – one to hold the shower and placate a frightened old lady, one to wash and the third to dry them and help them get dressed.

Older people often eat and drink poorly and are inactive. This can affect their digestive systems, resulting in constipation and incontinence. I don't remember diet being considered too much – there was certainly no restriction on the intake of chocolate Brazil nuts! But there were a variety of medicines to encourage working bowels. We did not resort to the weekly ritual that Jane encountered at one hospital in which she worked in the late 1980s; Friday morning meant 'bowel care' and all the patients were given an enema and sat on commodes facing each other in a circle.

At St Matthew's, once the routine of washing and dressing was complete, the ladies had nothing more to do than sit in the day room in an archetypal circle with the television occasionally on in the corner. Those likely to escape were pinned into their chairs by a tray that bolted across the front, rather like a high chair; quite rightly, these are banned today.

My friend Anne-Marie brought in a cassette radio and played a tape of 1940s songs, leading a singsong which the women thoroughly enjoyed. I wish I'd had her confidence. The permanent ward staff were thrilled – as if they had forgotten that they too could entertain their long-term charges.

It was Anne-Marie who persuaded me to take up my place at St Bartholomew's Hospital. My heart was set on college and journalism but she persuaded me it would be three years of fun. I could also see the valuable life experience that nursing would offer to a would-be writer. That, and it would please my mother.

As the offspring of a doctor and nurse parentage (and grand-parentage), there was little escape from the trajectory on which my brothers and I found ourselves. That we should all end up at the same hospital for the same three years, at the family alma mater, felt pre-determined. They as medical students, me as a student nurse.

Similarly, Caroline, who also comes from a comprehensively medical/nursing family, felt almost 'compelled' to do nursing from a very early age.

> I was given a nurse's uniform at about age three or four, and from then on it didn't occur to me to do anything else other than nursing. In my early teens I did consider medicine briefly but rapidly realised that I didn't have the brains or application to study that hard! I also had this romantic idea about nursing and the pretty uniforms.

Nursing, teaching and secretarial work were the employment destination for generations of women throughout the twentieth century. At one time nursing was about the only way that young women could leave home, have somewhere to live and earn an income, exchanging (often unwittingly) a suffocating home life for the excessive discipline of nurse training.

To Ruby, a 94-year-old former fever nurse, nursing represented every young girl's dream just as it did for Caroline, a generation or so later. She had worked in a munitions factory and hated it; her father didn't want her to go into the forces, so she was able to follow her dream of becoming a nurse. She did two years at Old Sarum Isolation Hospital before matron recommended her for SEN training which she completed at Ham Green Hospital, Bristol.

While it may be a childhood dream for some, there are also plenty who take up nursing almost by accident. For, as Dr Natalie Doyle, nurse consultant at the Royal Marsden NHS Foundation Trust, London, says, her friends were going off to university and she wondered what she would do. 'In the end, my Mum took charge and suggested I be a nurse.'

Natalie says the practicality of nursing, and later the opportunity she had to study and so contribute to an improvement in patient care, was incredibly rewarding. There are all kinds of nurses, she says: you can be with patients on the wards or in the community; you can be academic or political, influencing policy for the better of the profession and ultimately patients.

Less interested in how I would influence nursing and more in how nursing would influence me, my mother's unexpressed hope was that I would meet and marry the right calibre of man – a doctor obviously. After all, what had worked for her was surely right for me. I can report that despite some lame effort on the romance side, I entirely failed in this department. My brothers did much better. Both are doctors married to nurses and each has a child who is a doctor. Both my sisters-in-law are the daughters of doctors, with one, Elizabeth, the daughter of a doctor and nurse/midwife.

My father was the son of a doctor and nurse, and his sister, Molly, was also a nurse and midwife. My grandparents met on a fever ward in south London. She the redhaired petite ward sister, he the dashing young French doctor who later went on to teach and write textbooks on infectious diseases and was part of the team researching a vaccine against diphtheria. The experience of seeing young children on the infectious disease wards requiring tracheostomies and sometimes dying from diphtheria drove him on.

My grandmother, who was also a midwife, opened The Grange nursing home in Wimbledon – a maternity home for women giving birth. Pre-NHS days, couples paid a small amount each week during a woman's pregnancy towards the cost of being delivered in the comfort and safety of the nursing home. It was here that my father and his sister were brought up, mixing with the nursing staff and the elderly patients who were also catered for on the top floor of The Grange.

My parents met at St Bartholomew's Hospital in the 1950s; he a bright medical student who spent too much time producing the annual Hospital Revues and playing the piano in local pubs, she qualified, and nursed in New York for a year before returning to marry and bring up a family of would-be doctors and nurses. St Bartholomew's Hospital also played cupid to my older brother, while my other brother travelled all the way to South London where he met Mary Anne, a second-year student nurse at St Thomas's Hospital.

4

Part of his education as a medical student was to spend a week as a nursing auxiliary (care support worker). He presented for duty on Phipps ward at the South Western Hospital, home to mostly long-stay patients who had conditions such as polio, Guillain-Barré syndrome and motor neurone disease. Many of them were nursed in iron lungs, which are negative pressure ventilators helping people to breathe when their chest muscles no longer work.

All staff had to try out an iron lung so they could understand how they worked and what patients experienced, so later that day brother Stephen found himself in an iron lung. A typical test is to get the patient to count from one and as the machine forces them to take a breath so they are unable to make any sound although you can see them mouth the numbers, then as the machine relaxes so they can make a sound again. Mary Anne jokes: 'You could say I took his breath away on the first day we met!'

For them the rest is history. Romances that blossom within hospital often work because each understands that world, the extreme highs and lows and the overwhelming hours and demand.

For Caroline, who trained as a nurse and married a GP, this was certainly the case. Her brother and sister are both doctors, one married to a nurse, one to a doctor, while their parents met at medical school. It is who you meet, she says, as well as the common understanding of what the job involves. 'The horrors that we saw day to day at work creates a certain bond and puts you in a sort of "club" I think where you have a lot in common.'

For a long time, marriage was a bar to nursing. If you married you had to leave the job. There are many stories of (female) nurses who kept their marriage secret from their employer. It's not clear if this stemmed from society's belief that married women of a certain status shouldn't work, because nurses were expected to 'live-in' at the hospital and men were not allowed in the nurses' home, or whether it was a leftover from religious orders when nuns were married to God. Were nurses married to their patients? For many years, it appeared so, as so much was demanded of them and they had very little time off.

For a long time, especially post First World War, ward sisters were single women who stayed in the job for a lifetime, living in rooms just off the ward. In part this reflects an era when a generation of young men had been decimated by the war and by the 1918 'flu epidemic.

There were many single women needing a home and to earn a living. The Second World War increased the opportunities for work, although often nurses had little choice whether they would be deployed on the home front, which was in need of nurses and midwives in particular, or abroad as many wanted.

Changes in the demography of nurses came slowly after the Second World War, with unmarried, young, white females still predominating. Male nurses held sway in mental health nursing but there were few in general nursing, many of whom were thought to be gay for no other reason than they had taken up a caring profession.

Rob, who trained in the 1980s and met his future wife Jane, also a student nurse, says he was accosted in the street while in uniform by an 8-year-old boy announcing that he must be a 'poof'. Rob and Jane met, as nurses so often do, over the bedpan washer. Jane, who was a year ahead of him and therefore considerably more senior, had recruited his help to try and retrieve a set of false teeth she had thrown into the washer, buried as they were in a steel bowl full of vomit. Their attempts to recover the false teeth attracted the attention of the ward sister who wrenched open the bedpan washer in full flow, soaking herself as it belched steam at her. From this inauspicious start, romance blossomed for Rob and Jane.

Michael, whose wife Patience is also a nurse, did the combined mental health and general nursing course in the 1960s. He says that there were just three men in his set who came through the training. St Bartholomew's Hospital didn't accept a man onto its nurse training until 1979.

In the past, requirements to enter nursing could be fairly bizarre. Anything from the quality of your needlework skills to five 'O' levels and two 'A' levels, to references from a reverend. At one time, St Thomas's Hospital required references from three ministers of religion. Some schools might require you to write an essay about why you wanted to be a nurse, for others you needed to have done some voluntary work.

Your father's occupation was often important. There is no doubt that my family heritage weighed in my favour sufficiently, perhaps, to overlook the absence of a Maths 'O' level, but impossible for people who just didn't know their father, like Professor Dame Elizabeth Anionwu, who went on to be a leading advocate in the field of sickle cell screening and nursing. Dame Elizabeth says nursing schools also required that you send in a photograph of yourself.

Christine Hancock, who rose to be general secretary of the Royal College of Nursing, said her parents were told not to let her throw her life away on being a nurse, but if she did to be sure she went to Guy's Hospital, London. She recounts: 'Guy's asked a whole load of questions about my father. I wrote on the form that my father didn't want to be a nurse.' Christine went to King's College London.

Ann Keen, former Minister for Health, says she left school knowing all the words of John Lennon's songs but was not qualified in much else. Her first job working in a loo-roll factory checking the perforations in the paper did not increase her chances of being a nurse either, but a subsequent job as a receptionist in a casualty department brought Ann to the attention of one of the sisters who suggested she try for nurse training. Ann had to sit a General Nursing Council entry test – the so-called DC test – named after its author Dennis Child. Ann says she passed by one mark and was allowed to do the three year SRN course, although at the time she had no idea there were two tiers of entry to nursing.

Like most student nurses, Ann occasionally struggled with the excessive discipline. At 26, she was older than most of her contemporaries so when she saw her tiny room with the blankets folded on top of the mattress, the floppy white hat and collar stud, she felt she had joined the army.

Military style obedience was long considered a key requirement of nurses, especially students. Millicent Ashdown in her 1940s textbook says: 'A nurse must be punctual, good tempered, obedient and loyal to all rules.... They must ever remember that discipline and obedience are the keynote to satisfactory work in life; for to rule well we must first learn to obey.'

Doing not thinking

For most of the twentieth century, nurses trained through an apprenticeship model. We learned to 'do' rather than 'think', to conform rather than question. Our training was based on a medical model of curing illness and from this grew the conventional role of the nurse supporting the doctor, with little independent professional knowledge. It was a stereotype that was reinforced by the control doctors had over medical knowledge and how much of that was imparted to nurses in their training and in relation to the patients they nursed. Over the decades a more relaxed model evolved from the 'handmaiden' view of nurses to one of independent practice, but it was only when the nursing apprenticeship model came to an end that there was real change.

As students we were paid members of the ward team and there was a strict hierarchical system in place with new recruits at the bottom of the pile. On her first day in preliminary training school, Linda and her set were addressed by the Manchester Royal Infirmary school principal:

> She told us 'you are the lowest of the low'. I think most of us were quite surprised to hear this, however as we became more aware of the hierarchical system of nursing, in place at that time, we realised that indeed we were the lowest of the low and became adept at sliding under doors, pressing ourselves against the wall to make room for important individuals and hiding in the sluice.

The training worked on a system of ward placements interspersed with a block of teaching – two weeks in the classroom and then onto a new ward. In previous eras, nurses had to attend classes in their own time, running (well, walking quickly) straight from a long shift on the ward to lectures given by doctors. This approach was often based on learning by rote, usually at the hands of a more senior nurse, and led to an almost formulaic set of skills for any given situation.

'Doing not thinking', was how Virginia Henderson described it, as quoted in the preface of this book. To challenge anything upset the order of things, and good order was the very backbone of good nursing and the bedrock of rituals.

Good order and non-questioning made running a ward easier. According to the seminal work by Menzies Lyth, *Social Systems as a Defence against Anxiety* in the 1960s, the task orientated ritualistic nature of nursing work was a way of nurses managing the anxiety they felt in the face of constant physical and mental distress among their patients.

This depersonalisation, as Menzies Lyth describes it, worked two ways. Patients were (and often still are) referred to as 'bed five', or 'the hernia in bed six'. Avoiding a personal relationship with patients while providing a deeply personal service enabled nurses to deal with a stressful and distressing job by avoiding any emotional attachment.

Such depersonalisation helped to smooth out any individuality of nurse or patient: all patients had to behave in a certain way and accept their role as patients, while nurses were indistinguishable from each other.

Michael recounts how, on a consultant ward round on the psychogeriatric ward where he worked, he called one of the patients by their first name, knowing the patient would not respond to anything more formal. The consultant, wishing not to be overheard, took Michael aside to an open window where, speaking out into the open air, he admonished him for using the patient's first name.

When I began training, twenty years later, we were warned that we were not to let patients know our first names. We were always 'Nurse Smith' or whatever. On my first ward I stood my ground, all red-faced, refusing to tell one patient my first name. Naturally I discovered later that none of my friends kept this ridiculous rule!

At the same time, Fay was working across London in a coronary care unit where they brought in the practice of patients calling them by their first names. She says it was regarded as revolutionary.

Procedure book

On every ward we relied on a procedure book – a hefty A4 file stored in the treatment room to which we could hastily refer when asked to carry out an unfamiliar procedure. The processes described were rarely based on scientific research or evidence of effectiveness, but on the express preferences of the consultants or ward sister. In Tom's day, students created their own procedure books, adding to the file as they learned new procedures, helping them tick off the competencies they were required to learn on each ward and providing them with a veritable bible for their future practice, but also risking perpetuating poor or outdated processes.

When I did a return to practice course in the early 2000s, all of us had trained under the old system and were nonplussed at the absence of a procedure book. It meant we had to think! Modern nurses apply their knowledge and experience and take action. No need for comforting, procedure books. In recent years, the word 'protocol' has become popular and there are protocols for all kinds of care – managing a significant drop in blood sugar or a haemorrhage, for instance.

These are vital and it means everyone understands what to do in a crisis – so procedure has its place – providing it is evidence based.

The move away from apprenticeship nurse training came in 1986 with the introduction of Project 2000 (P2K). P2K was about health not illness and the first eighteen months were theoretical – triple that of the traditional courses – and the students were supernumerary, no longer a part of the workforce.

Erica trained on the P2K programme in 1990. She says she and her fellow students were taught to question – maybe the first generation of nurses to be so encouraged. 'They [the tutors] were trying to shift the goalposts so you had an inquiring mind and evidence based practice.'

Erica says they were also told to not work in a ritualistic manner, which could be challenging and was not always welcomed on traditional wards: 'We were wet behind the ears, what did we know?'

It was a difficult transition for everyone. New nursing students often found it difficult to reconcile what they were learning in the classroom with what they were expected to do on the wards. A lack of practical training was keenly felt. Michael, who was an educator on the new training course says more thought should have been given to the students' expectations of a nursing course, which were still fairly traditional.

Caroline, who like Michael had trained under the apprenticeship model of nursing, also taught on Project 2000. She says: 'I was teaching nursing when P2K came out, so had experience of the "before and after". At the time I felt strongly that the new style of training left newly qualified staff nurses ill prepared for the role.'

Nursing has to be a scientifically aware, evidence-based profession and it is right that it is now a profession that requires a degree – just like physiotherapy or occupational therapy – but many people think this affects nurses' ability to be compassionate and caring. So much so that in 2012, the chief nursing officer set out a vision for nursing called Compassion in Practice, more commonly referred to as the 6 Cs: Care, Compassion, Competence, Communication, Courage and Commitment – to reinforce the values required of people wanting to do nursing and to meet the expectations of the public.

Associate nurses have very recently completed their first courses – two-year apprenticeship style training – and they will fill a gap between HCAs and registered nurses, similar to the enrolled nurse that was such a vital part of the nursing workforce for the best part of forty years.

Some would argue that now the role of students on the wards has been taken over by health care assistants (HCAs), also known as care support workers (CSWs), it is they who provide the bulk of physical care, the tasks of bed baths and bed pans, with staff nurses managing the ward, coordinating the care, the admissions and discharges, the drug rounds and the technical demands.

Tasks tend to lead to routines: 'the washes, the obs, the drugs', rather than individualised care. There is no doubt that routine provides structure which is comforting to both nurses and patients. The risk is that routines become rituals – the routine becoming an end in itself which led to some unusual practices in the past – and is may be creating some modern day ones that we don't yet recognise.

Chapter 2

Nurses Who Rustle

'Nurses should always remember the sacredness of their profession, and hold it in such respect that they will never bring discredit on their uniform.'

Confronted by the uniform laid out on the bed in the tiny room in the nurses' home, together with a square of starched linen to be made into a hat, I recognised my first challenge as a student nurse. Making a hat remained a hurdle for the next three years.

The idea was that the linen square was laid over a round biscuit tin – a shortbread tin seemed to be first choice – and pleats were made on each side and somehow two dove tails were pulled through and folded over the top and held together with a series of grips. To my teenage embarrassment, my mother, previously a Bart's nurse, fashioned a hat for me there and then. Unfortunately, there was a generational difference in style between the 1950s and the 1980s, and while my tutors applauded 'my' efforts, my new fellow students sniggered and made smart hats for themselves.

Susie, who confesses to choosing Bart's because she liked the uniform best, arrived with a hat ready-made:

> I knew someone at Bart's and she made me a hat on a biscuit tin before I started, so I paid little attention to how to make them and wore the original one for months. I used to get someone to make me one every time I needed a new one.

Through three years, I stifled my growing concern that my hat, refreshed and renewed only occasionally, was more likely to be an infection risk than a preventive measure.

Hats were not simply coverings for the hair, preventing the transmission of bacteria from patient to patient or even, in Victorian times, as a method of exposing possible infestation of headlice picked out against the white of the hat. Hats were handy for hiding cigarettes: Linda who trained in the 1960s says:

> Morning tea was when we learned how fast we could walk.
> No running allowed. We had fifteen minutes to walk to
> the dining room, down tea/coffee, and biscuits and most
> importantly have at least three puffs of a cigarette. No time
> to finish it so cut off the end neatly with scissors and place
> in front fold of cap for safe keeping.

Hats were part of the hierarchy. Most nursing schools had their own designs and all kinds of status was accorded to them depending on the height of the hat and whether it had ribbons and frills.

In *Patients Come First,* Margaret Broadley describes the elaborate cap bestowed on her when she became a sister in the 1920s: 'The cap was made up of three pieces; a top, consisting of a double row of gophered lace frills, from which were suspended two similarly decorated waist length tails.'

Leaping up to respond to doctors appearing for a ward round, Margaret caught her 'tails' between a bed screen and the chair. Not noticing the tug of her hair pins as the stiffly starched cap was pulled from her head and stood suspended mid-air, she made a stately bareheaded progression down the ward.

A generation later, Jan remembers how proud she felt when matron presented with her staff nurse's hat, glancing at her reflection and feeling the bounce of the starched peak as she walked down the corridor back to the ward. The hat itself was completely inappropriate for the practicalities of nursing.

Similarly, nurses at Bart's who reached their fifth year of service wore a 'fifth year cap'. This was white starched muslin set in a small peak and was a short version of a sister's longer cap. It invariably got knocked off or caught in the curtains when helping to move a patient in the small space around a patient's bed. Keeping it starched and upright was quite a skill, achieved by the insertion of cardboard – from a cereal packet or a patient X-ray card, which were just the right size.

Hats are emblematic of nursing and were discarded with great reluctance by many at the end of the twentieth century as the profession tore itself away from an old-fashioned culture rooted in its own rituals and myths. Jane Salvage in her book *The Politics of Nursing*, says that hats were the last vestige of the veil and symbolised 'modesty and obedience'.

Religious orders were among the first to offer nursing care and this, together with a strong nod to the servant classes mixed with Florence Nightingale's military influence from the Crimea, led to an early uniform of plain dresses, starched aprons, cloaks with the famous red straps across the front, all with silver badges and buckles.

Queen Victoria, who had taken a keen interest in Florence's work in Crimea was a valuable ally as Florence strove to establish nursing as a profession in the UK. Together, with other leading ladies of the day they took some eighteen months to come up with the design for a uniform that would put a distance between Charles Dickens's 'Sairey Gamp' image of nurses and what Florence had in mind. Sairey Gamp is a nurse in *Martin Chuzzlewit*, described as dissolute, sloppy and generally drunk. Florence and co. wanted the image of nurses to be clean, educated and demure – something akin to the top of the servant hierarchy.

Florence was influenced by the uniforms worn by the Deaconesses at Kaiserworth in Germany, where she visited at the start of her nursing mission. The deaconesses' clothes were plain blue cotton gowns with a white apron, a large turned down collar and a white muslin cap with a frill around the face, tied with a large bow beneath the chin. It's thought this description of a uniform worn in a caring role is one of the earliest recorded. It is remarkably similar to the nurses' uniforms of much of the twentieth century, give or take changes in hem length, hats and fabric.

For a design so long in development, you would have hoped they might have come up with something more practical than white aprons and dresses that were difficult to move in. The predominance of white had its roots in employers being able to check their servants were carrying out their laundry at suitable intervals. Indeed, having a clean apron was one of the essentials of being a nurse for the next eighty years.

Modesty was considered more important than practicality. Modesty mirrored the feminine myth that nurses, like all women, should be demure and diffident. Describing uniform in her seminal text *Notes on Nursing: what it is and what it is not*, Florence commented that patients were 'repulsed' by 'nurses who rustle'. Adding, 'The fidget of silk and crinoline, the rattling of keys, the creaking of stays and of shoes, will do a patient more harm than all the medicines in the world will do him good.'

Much importance was attached to appearance as described by Millicent Ashdown: 'A nurse must be ... careful to wear her uniform with spotless cleanliness, neatness and simplicity ... her general bearing that of military smartness.'

There is many a nurse who remembers the supposed impropriety of wearing sleeves (removable white cuffs) for the wrong task or worse still, speaking to a doctor when not wearing sleeves. Margaret Broadley says that at the London Hospital in the 1920s, later the Royal London Hospital, sleeves were worn for serving meals and giving medicines, and taken off when carrying out any form of treatment. To speak to a doctor when not wearing sleeves was a 'heinous offence'.

Ruby says that even when nurses were in the sluice up to their elbows in rinsing out nappies on the children's infectious diseases ward, if matron was on a ward round, you had to remove your rubber gloves, roll down your sleeves, pull the cuff frills on and stand by the sluice door until matron had gone past. Then off with the cuffs, up with the sleeves and back on with the rubber gloves.

At St Bartholomew's Hospital in the 1920s and 1930s, sleeves were long, with an opening extending not less than 6 inches from the wrist and fastened with six buttons. At the wrist there was a detachable cuff, 2½ inches wide, which was worn to serve food, for officially speaking to sister (I'm not sure there was any unofficial speaking to sister) or for leaving the ward. While working in the wards, nurses were expected to put their cuffs in their pocket and roll up their sleeves.

In the 1980s Susie yearned to be a Pink (junior sister at Bart's) simply because of the glamorous pale pink uniform with long sleeves (frowned upon now) and accompanying Pink's basket. The Pink's basket was left over from previous eras when all nurses at the hospital were given baskets in which they carried their clean aprons for putting on after coffee when the dirty work of the ward was done and the dressings would start. It was also handy for smokers to pop their cigarettes in.

Linda trained at Manchester Royal Infirmary. The uniform was a short sleeved green dress with button-on starched white collar and cuffs. She says:

> It had a starched white apron the bib of which reached to the collar of the dress, wide straps were crossed over one's back and brought around the waist to be secured by a safety pin at the front. The apron's waist band was then buttoned at the back thus covering most of the dress. The uniform had to be exactly eleven inches from the ground. A white starched cap was folded into shape and secured on the head with white Kirby grips. The shoes were heavy brown lace ups and we wore brown stockings with seams at the back which had always to be straight.

The seniority of nursing was depicted by adding two white stripes onto the right sleeve of the uniform for the second year and a third stripe to depict third year status.

> After passing our final SRN exams we were staff nurses and entitled to wear 'strings' and a green belt. The strings were two strips of starched white material, the ends of which we fashioned into a very complicated bow. This was worn under the chin and the ends went up behind the ears and were tied on the top of our heads then secured with Kirby grips. The cap was placed over them. The strings were incredibly uncomfortable but we wore them with pride.

Ann, who trained in London in the late 1960s, describes the hierarchy's obsession with the length and cut of the uniform. A group of nurses had raised money for charity and she and a few friends had been nominated to give the money to Princess Margaret at a performance of the musical, *Hello Dolly.*

> For some reason we were to go in uniform although usually you weren't allowed outside the hospital in uniform. We went to matron's office where she had us standing on the table so she could measure us from the hem of our uniform

dresses to ankle to ensure it was the correct length and that not too much leg was exposed. She also checked that no more than an inch and a half of hair was poking out from our hats.

We arrived at the theatre with its red carpet outside and as we walked up the stairs someone had a heart attack in front of us. None of us knew what to do as we hadn't done heart attacks in our training yet and this sort of incident was the whole reason we didn't go out in uniform. The upshot was we never met Princess Margaret, we never handed over the money and we didn't see the musical!

The fate of the man who had the heart attack can only be guessed at.

Uniform presents a powerful symbol of professionalism; something that public and other healthcare professionals can instantly recognise and be reassured by. On the other hand, there are those who think that it depersonalises and anonymises people and is a way of a hospital maintaining control over the nursing profession. Some have described uniform as part of a medical model of nursing.

White coats are no longer worn by doctors, ties are forbidden (unless of the bow variety and that raises a whole other set of questions) and no shirt cuffs – 'bare below the elbows' – as part of controlling the risk of infection-spread. Uniform has not been worn in mental health settings for nearly fifty years. But for general nurses, the direct contact with bodily fluids swings it for me. I would rather wear clothes on the ward that I wouldn't wear for anything else – whether it be scrubs or tunic and trousers.

With the advent of the NHS a 'national' uniform was introduced but was never universally adopted, with the big teaching hospitals continuing to have their own uniforms. Some did adopt the blue and white check dress but the fabric was cheap and it was not well liked.

Some leading hospitals recruited famous fashion designers to bring style and comfort to their staff. Queen Mary was president of the London Hospital and in the 1940s, Norman Hartnell, fashion designer to the royals, was commissioned to design the London Hospital nurses' uniform. The dresses had puffed sleeves, pearl buttons down the front and a large pleat at the back to allow for stretching. Every nurse was fitted for a bespoke uniform. Recalling the uniform in *Nursing Through the Years: care and compassion at the Royal London Hospital,* Marjorie says it was the most comfortable uniform she ever wore.

In *Politics of Nursing*, Jane Salvage reports on a 1980 *Nursing Times* competition for readers to design a 'uniform fit for the 80s'. Favourites were traditional dresses and caps. The winner commented that her design: 'reintroduced into the uniform the femininity which most nurses feel has been lost'.

One wonders what the men who were nurses made of that.

In 2006, fashion designer Paul Costelloe designed new uniforms for the nurses of Guy's and St Thomas's Hospital, London. At the time, every nurse in the Trust was measured to make sure that the new uniforms fitted perfectly. There was not much change to the traditional uniform style but the idea was that patients would recognise who were nurses and who were not. As to the different colours for different ranks that is still a lingering reminder of the military need for keeping order and hierarchy.

Very often these days, both nurses and doctors are in scrubs – they are comfortable and functional and it does away with some of that hierarchy. However, it can leave the patient unsure who they are talking to. The 'hello my name is' campaign was created by Dr Kate Granger MBE, a registrar in elderly care medicine who had terminal cancer. Dr Granger started the campaign in August 2013 after she became frustrated with staff who failed to introduce themselves to her when she was a patient. Kate used social media to help kick start the campaign and created the hashtag #hellomynameis. Kate died in 2016 but her legacy continues.

Based in the City of London, St Bartholomew's Hospital is flanked by St Paul's Cathedral, the Old Bailey and Smithfield meat market. I remember the raucous atmosphere in the meat market as I walked through its great arches after night duty. The pubs would be open and serving beer alongside huge breakfasts and many hospital staff took the opportunity to call in on their way home. All the meat men wore white coats, which seemed something of an odd proximity to a large hospital where the doctors still wore white coats.

In her first year, Paula was startled by the appearance at the ward door of a man wearing a white coat spattered with blood. Assuming he was a porter from the meat market, she told him in no uncertain terms that he couldn't enter the ward as it was not visiting time. She was mortified when he informed her that he was professor of medicine and consultant to the ward.

It was also possible at Bart's to mistake the visiting barber for a doctor, as he too wore a white coat, which given that surgeons were originally barbers doesn't seem entirely inappropriate. The barber would provide those shaves for the men that might otherwise be embarrassing for a young female nurse to perform. There was no such delicacy at Hackney Hospital where we did half of our training. There, nipple to groin shaves for almost every kind of abdominal surgery was standard. And body hair is so hard to shift. I remember getting all kinds of flustered trying to shave a poor man awaiting a cholecystectomy (removal of gall bladder). My friends Jackie and Margaret recount doing a groin shave for a man, which for some reason took two of them amid lots of stifled giggling.

Badges and Buckles

From the earliest days of nursing right through to when nursing schools moved into universities and adopted their logos and culture, badges have been a treasured part of becoming a registered nurse. The badges have become collectors' items as very few universities award them and their value, both fiscal and sentimental, has increased.

The Victorians loved medals and decorations and as far back as the 1860s these were awarded to encourage higher standards. Many of the nursing badges have their origins in military, chivalric and religious orders. Some carry symbols of vigilance (the crane) or self-sacrifice (the pelican) The latter features on the Royal Infirmary Edinburgh School of Nursing badge. It depicts a pelican sitting on her nest and plucking her breast to feed her young with her blood, symbolising the nurse's dedication to the service of others. Holders of the RIE School of Nursing or RIE Enrolled Nurse (EN) Training School badge came to be known as 'Pelicans'.

Animals and flowers feature. The Simpson Memorial Maternity Pavilion (a maternity hospital incorporated in the RIE), badge had a butterfly at the centre. The pomegranate, as seen on the early Royal College of Midwives badge, represents fertility, while snowdrops on the Glasgow Royal Maternity badge are for motherhood. Badges gained in maternity tend to be round so there are no sharp edges to harm the baby when the midwife picks it up. The Glasgow Royal Infirmary School of Nursing featured three thistle heads on a staff and a serpent entwined, representing the serpent-entwined rod of healing with the inscription: 'Auspice Caelo', which is also found on the wall of Glasgow Royal Infirmary on Castle Street. Translated it means, 'By the favour of heaven'.

There are numerous badges associated with the armed services and nursing. Many of them designed to look like medals, while the intricacy of the work is beautiful. Anyone who has attended the Florence Nightingale memorial service held every May on Florence's birthday in Westminster Abbey could not fail to be impressed by the ranks of nursing military represented there in full uniform, chests adorned with medals and badges.

Nurses are immensely proud of their training school and proud to wear the badge. As Linda remembers of her training at Manchester Royal Infirmary:

> After a year as a staff nurse and having completed our hospital exams we were presented with a bronze belt and the Manchester Royal Infirmary Hospital Badge. A large round bronze badge depicting the Good Samaritan with the words 'Vade et tu fac' similiter engraved around the edge. 'Go and do thou likewise'. Our badge or Penny, as we called it, was worn on the right side of our apron and we were now Senior Staff Nurses. We were and I still am, extremely proud of the Manchester Royal Infirmary Penny.

The design of the badge of the Nightingale Training School was taken from the eight-pointed cross of the Knights of the Hospital of St John of Jerusalem. Its four arms symbolise the Cardinal Virtues – Prudence, Temperance, Justice and Fortitude.

The black-and-white Wakering shield has been St Bartholomew's Hospital badge for more than 500 years. The design is taken from the Coat of Arms used by John Wakering, who was the Master of the Hospital from 1423 to 1462.

Local industry or hospital benefactors were sometimes behind the design of hospital badges or buckles. The badge for the Princess Margaret Hospital, Swindon, has a train at the centre of it – Swindon being on the route of The Great Western Trains with a huge rail industry. The hospital was officially opened by Princess Margaret in 1966 but has since been demolished and replaced by the Great Western Hospital.

The London Hospital's badge was particularly impressive: designed to be pinned to the uniform and hang like a military medal, it was a heavy Maltese cross with four fleur-de-leys in each corner, hanging from a red and blue ribbon. It is rumoured that the bronze metal was from a cannon captured in the Crimean war. The ribbon is supposedly from the Colonel in Chief of the Household Brigade who was thrown from his horse and taken to the hospital. To show his gratitude for his nursing care, he asked Queen Victoria for the right of nurses at the hospital to wear the ribbon of the regiment.

Other training schools had badges that reflected their courses. For instance, the Oxford Eye Hospital badge is designed to look like an eye, and for nurses who trained at the former Southampton Eye Hospital – there is now an Eye Unit of Southampton General Hospital – the badge shows a symbolic eagle with drops of red enamel. The red enamel is the heraldic representation for surgery and the eagle is a reference to the legendary eyesight of birds of prey.

Following Ethel Gordon Fenwick's successful campaign for the Nurses Registration Act of 1919, the General Nursing Council (GNC) of England and Wales, with separate GNCs of Scotland and Ireland were established. The Councils' role was to compile and maintain a register of qualified nurses, and to act as the disciplinary authority of the profession. The State General Nursing Council (GNC) badge with its blue border was introduced in 1922 and in the 1940s the SEN badge, with its green border came into being for England & Wales. It was awarded to nurses when they registered.

The GNC was one of the nine bodies replaced on 30 June 1983 by the United Kingdom Central Council for Nursing, Midwifery and Health Visiting (UKCC) and subsequently replaced again by the Nursing and Midwifery Council (NMC). That time is etched in my memory as it coincided (almost to the day) with my qualifying as a nurse and suddenly I was no longer going to be a State Registered Nurse (SRN) as it then was in England, but a Registered General Nurse (RGN) – a title that had been in place for many years in Scotland. At the time I felt I had been cheated. In some ways I had, for the UKCC declared it would not be issuing badges to newly qualified nurses. This may have had something to do with the fact that there were by then some 750,000 names on the Register (for RGNs) and Roll (for ENs). It may also have been an honest attempt to move away from the sentimentality of nurses with hats and frills and accessories to one of professionals without need for adornment. I was still miffed.

Belt buckles were another source of uniform pride to nurses when they qualified or 'belted'. There was, of course a particular colour belt usually made of petersham, to indicate qualification – often, but not always, navy blue – which was clasped at the waist with a silver buckle. Some of the teaching hospitals produced their own buckle with the hospital badge at the centre. St Bartholomew's Hospital had the Wakering Shield, while University College Hospital had a maple leaf, a nod to one of its sponsors – a local maple furniture shop. The Westminster Hospital buckle featured a central motif of the Portcullis design of the nearby Palace of Westminster. Buckles finally went out for good in the 1990s because they were cited as an infection and/or patient hazard risk, although it's not clear how many patients have been injured by a nurses' buckle (the image is not a good one), or whether buckles were ever actually tested as harbingers of infection.

Accessories

Over the course of our training we would add small status symbols to our uniform. For example, attaching a cord clamp to scissors after doing the midwifery placement – useful for clamping the call bell to a patient's bed sheet in the years before call bell clamps came as standard. A wooden tongue depressor with the formulae for the number of drops per minute required for different intravenous infusion rates was an absolute necessity and crept into a nurse's top pocket probably after completion of the drug assessment.

A set of Spencer Wells forceps were a key part of any self-respecting nurse's accoutrements. Used for anything from tapping the tubing on an intravenous drip to make bubbles disappear, to rather viciously twisting the same tubing around the forceps to somehow encourage infusion flow. This was a ritual I associated with being a staff nurse who could solve anything. I recognise it now as both bad practice and a ritual that rarely worked. Alexandra, ITU nurse, says Spencer Wells are still good for undoing Luer locks on infusions or for connecting infusions to central venous catheters.

In A&E, Gail remembers carrying curved Mayo scissors, a must for trimming plaster of Paris casts, and what she describes as 'big vicious scissors' for cutting off clothes. Everything was labelled with baby name tags – written cards inside plastic – to stop them ending up in the wrong pockets. There's many a nurse who has kept their Spencer Wells for several decades – so handy for any number of DIY jobs from unscrewing tops off jars to extracting hair from bath plugs.

For Kayte, training just a few years later in 1990, hats and aprons had gone and all the aspiring nurse had about her person were a watch, a pen and a stethoscope. A stethoscope! The very symbol of knowing what you are doing. For the best part of my nursing life, you could borrow a ward stethoscope to listen to blood pressures on the ancient sphygmomanometers, having first cleaned the ear buds with alcohol wipes. I'm searching my memory to know what we cleaned them with before alcohol wipes were invented and slightly sickeningly, I can't remember…

Chapter 3

Handover and Hierarchy

'We had a consultant who wanted all his patients on the bed, underwear off and covered with a blanket for his ward round.'

The consultant ward round was the big event of the day. Each consultant had his (almost always his) own peculiar rituals. This might include how the ward was to look, where the nurses were meant to be (usually in the sluice, apart from the ward sister), whether the patients were under the covers or on top, indeed whether the patient was actually spoken to or just spoken about.

At about bed 19 there was the customary nod from sister to a junior nurse to go and put the kettle on so tea was ready for the great man at the end of the round, when sister would deploy her best china to entertain him in her office. Linda trained at the MRI in the 1960s:

> The ward must be tidy, beds made, bed wheels turned in, curtains back and all patients sitting up in bed, preferably at the same angle. I think that it would have been acceptable to have run around with a feather duster flicking any sign of dust or imperfections from each patient prior to the Great Man's Arrival.

The consultant would make his entry followed by his entourage in white coats: registrar, houseman, medical students, to be greeted by sister who would accompany them on their round, pushing the notes trolley so that each patient's notes were to hand. Junior nurses were dispatched to the sluice.

Anne remembers one occasion when the ward round set off, consultant, sister and the entourage of doctors and medical students and, horrors! Sister's dress was caught in her knickers. Everyone froze.

Discreetly, the consultant drew her behind the curtains, advised her of the delicate matter and she emerged red-faced, smoothing her dress. Order was restored.

Still in introductory block, we students were allocated to a 'taster' day on the ward where we would spend our first three months. Jacqui was sent to female surgical. On the consultant's round her role was to hold a hot water bottle on two outstretched hands so he could warm his hands before examining a patient. The round was in full swing; all the patients were lying on top of their beds, arms by their sides, curtains pulled around the bed leaving the same width of opening at each bed, measured by a yardstick used solely for this purpose, to allow the great man access.

The bleep in the consultant's pocket sounded. He looked at the registrar and said 'answer that'. The registrar looked at the staff nurse and said 'answer that' and she looked at Jacqui, the most junior person present and said 'answer that'. Jacqui had no idea what a bleep was or how you answered it, but as the sound came from the consultant's trousers, she bent forward, still holding the hot water bottle on outstretched hands and yelled into his pocket 'hello, hello!' There was a stunned silence and then uproarious laughter. Jacqui was dismissed from the ward round. She says that many years later she met an obstetric consultant who relayed the now legendary story to her without realising that it was Jacqui's own.

Joy worked in women's health: 'We had a consultant who wanted all his patients on the bed, underwear off and covered with a blanket for his ward round.'

Knickers off and never mind the indignity, was quite a ritual in women's health and maternity. Jane says:

> When I was a midwife in part of the West Midlands it was custom and practice in that area for ladies in antenatal clinics after producing the regulation urine sample, to remove their underwear so time was not wasted by removing underwear when going to see doctor or midwife.

Similarly, Kathy reports that in the contraception clinics of the 1970s, women sat in the waiting room with their stockings around their ankles, just so they didn't take up any more of the doctor's time than was necessary.

These days medical students are taught communication skills and are much better at discussing treatment options with their patients and generally treating them as human beings. But it was not always so and there are recent reports of consultants who won't allow relatives to be present during consultations with patients. I suppose it stops them asking any questions!

There are still consultants who like to be treated as though they are gods and prefer to bark their orders, but they are less common than previously. As society has moved on, so this sort of behaviour is less tolerated.

At one time the consultant may not have spoken directly to the patient but rather about him or her with his colleagues, conferring at the end of the bed or speaking in loud tones as if the thin curtains around the bed provided some sort of sound barrier to the rest of the ward listening intently.

I worked on one women's health ward where the consultant stopped at the end of the bed of a young woman being treated for pelvic inflammatory disease, a condition often caused by sexually transmitted infection. He turned to his entourage and said in a voice not altogether sotto voce: 'Some men put their penises where I wouldn't put the tip of my umbrella.'

A few students sniggered – after all, this was the man who would write their references. No one dared challenge him

Sue says one consultant was asked by a patient whom he had sterilised how soon the operation would be effective, 'He told her to wait until she got home!'

The same consultant insisted on having an ashtray on the notes trolley for his ward round and used to sit in sister's office, feet up on the desk and flick the ash of his cigar into the sink.

> He was a biker and regularly did his rounds in his leathers.
> I once tried to chuck him off the ward when he came in his
> bike gear. He still had his helmet on and I thought he was a
> cheeky visitor trying to sneak in.

Nikki, a ward sister for many years says that the old ward round was one routine that hospitals should have kept. Prima-donna behaviour by consultants aside, it offered a team approach where the nursing staff, junior doctors and the patient all heard the same information and knew the treatment plan. These days, ward rounds happen at any time, and with fewer nurses, it is rare that anyone can be spared to accompany visiting doctors. Wards have expanded to become whole departments and may have upwards of fifteen or twenty consultants, so keeping up with all of them is impossible.

Chaperoning a male doctor while he examines a female patient is important for the safety and comfort of both doctor and patient. Kathy says that chaperoning should not mean also playing handmaiden to a doctor who wishes to be waited on, which for many decades was a ritual that each profession danced to. Chaperoning, she says, means being there to support the patient at the head end rather than the business end.

Then there is the chaperone who is not really there. In the 1950s at Bart's, female medical students were still something of a rarity, so when they presented at the staff sick rooms for their health examination prior to starting training, the examining doctor would telephone his secretary and say he was about to examine Miss Smith. He would then hand the phone to the prospective student who would stay in communication with the secretary – presumably female.

That some of the men – from porters to nurses to doctors – were given to thinking a pretty nurse was fair game was a reflection of how things were in wider society. All too often nurses in uniform were not necessarily thought of as people with feelings but as glamorous objects – not helped by the media's portrayal of nurses as angels or sex symbols. Mary Anne, newly appointed sister in ICU, was advised by her nursing officer that one of the consultants could be a 'bit handsy', so when he put his arm around her waist on the ward round, she extracted herself from his grasp and remained out of reach. At the end of the round she spoke to him alone telling him his behaviour was out of order. He was hugely apologetic and said no one had ever told him that before. The nursing officer, horrified that the consultant had been spoken to in this way, apologised to him on Mary Anne's behalf. But he said that Mary Anne was quite right and he was in the wrong. As far as she knew he did not behave inappropriately again to members of staff.

Alison, bent double underneath the sink in the theatre scrub room, cleaning up used paper towels, together with all the other items people had chucked at the bin and missed, when she felt a large hand on her rear. Thinking it was some silly trick being played by a fellow student or an operating department assistant with a warm-water filled glove she indignantly bellowed: 'Oh, go away! I'm busy and so unimpressed by this juvenile behaviour.'

There was a muffled grunt and as Alison stood up and whirled round, she caught sight of the bulky figure of the day's surgeon, making a rapid exit. Nowadays, says Alison, there would be uproar but then, in the 1980s, we just accepted that he was a renowned roué with wandering hands.

Escort duties

Not to be confused with any other kind of escort duties, escorting patients to another hospital is a ritual for which no savvy nurse willingly volunteers. Invariably the patient is more ill than you have been told, or at least the act of moving them has destabilised their condition. The journey and transfer take longer than anyone thought. The receiving ward is at best civil and at worst claims to have no idea you were coming. And it is an absolutely time-honoured fact that you will struggle to get home again. Transport will have 'just left', no one at the receiving end will care who you are or how you are going to get home, while the colleagues who you thought were your mates back on your own ward will have gone home for the day.

Debbie thought she had chosen an easy option when, working at Bart's, a call went out for a volunteer to escort a patient to Stanmore. As Stanmore was a ward at the end of the corridor she willingly offered, only to find herself in the back of an ambulance, very car sick, with a quadriplegic patient who had a tracheostomy – and so required intensive nursing care – as they trundled at 10 miles an hour all the way to the Royal National Orthopaedic Hospital in Stanmore – a good 15 miles away.

Rachael had to escort a patient to the German psychiatric hospital in Dalston, East London, from the observation ward at Bart's hospital. A short journey but she says:

> The only way to keep this patient calm was to give him sweets. So, before I got in the ambulance, I stuffed my pockets full of Quality Street raided from the ward tin. As we drove off, I kept smiling nicely and offering this patient a chocolate. Of course, he asked for more. I then told him I just had one left so he would need to eat it slowly.

On hearing this, the paramedic accompanying Rachael banged on the window to the driver saying: 'put the blues on she's running out of sweets.'

Rachael says: 'We belted through Hackney with all lights flashing and I handed the patient over... but not before mistaking the charge nurse for a psychiatric patient.'

In the mid-1970s, Judy was asked to escort a patient by train from London to a hospital on the south coast.

> I only had cash for my lunch and was stuck on one of those old fashioned trains with no corridor armed only with a male urinal in case the patient needed to pass urine. At the hospital the ambulance crew asked how I was getting back to the station. I had no idea where I was or how to get there and no money. They kindly took me back!

Lynne also remembers travelling by train, two nurses this time with a tea urn and a whole carriage full of patients looking forward to convalescence. 'Those were the days – three weeks in hospital post op then a week or so by the sea in a convalescent home – often union or works funded.'

Kathy worked at King's College Hospital in London and says the hospital had its own convalescent home in Camberley, Surrey, where grateful ladies were sent post-hysterectomy for a week's rest. 'Most of them had never been out of London before and they came back to see the consultant six weeks post op looking so rested'.

Wherever you work, you are convinced that your ward has it hardest, has fewest staff, has the most challenging patients. Therefore, in theory, handing over a patient from one ward to another represents more work for the receiving ward and less for you, often making it a tense process.

Worse, it is quite likely that the nurse handing over has not been looking after the patient but simply tasked with the job of transporting them, so knows nothing about them other than what she has been told in a breathless rush by a colleague. Whatever the situation, there is often a barely disguised rudeness from the receiving team that puts the handover person on the back foot. It maybe they have overlooked some small detail or there could be a minor discrepancy in the age, diagnosis or health status of the patient. Perhaps the patient has been brought earlier or later than expected. I've experienced this edginess when simply transferring a patient to theatre. Whatever it is there is some sort of triumphant 'told you so' behaviour from the receiving team should they detect a minor infringement that isn't especially friendly.

Report

Handover, or report, as it was known when I was a student, filled me with terror. As a self-conscious teenager, I hated being the centre of attention and was terrified of speaking in front of others. There were all kinds of rituals attached to report that I took a while to grasp. There was a hierarchy as to where you were allowed to sit. The most senior nurse (usually sister/charge nurse) would have the proper chair at the desk while the rest of us balanced ourselves on the footstools that were usually at the end of patients' beds, dragging them into a sort of semi-circle around the desk and arranging ourselves according to rank.

How to hand over was not taught in the classroom but learned by example on the ward so it was always ripe for ritual. Much of being a nurse is about modelling yourself on other nurses. This was particularly so in the days of apprenticeship nursing when much of the learning was done on the ward. We observed our colleagues, how they carried themselves, whether they were confident and used the correct terminology or whether they mumbled and blushed and forgot the important stuff (me).

Certainly, when I wasn't marvelling at the tilt of sister's hat or the pinkness of the junior sister's uniform, I was learning from their conduct, their questions and the concerns they voiced about patients. These tended to be the younger sisters. The old-school ones gave little away and too often used handover as a time to remind us of what we hadn't done rather than what we had (unless that was wrong too).

Handover is different everywhere so with every ward change you needed to learn quickly 'how it's done here'. When I was a student, your opinion counted for nothing but you were expected to know about your patients and be able to report what you had done for them and their state of health. Usually we carried little notebooks and quickly developed nursing shorthand and symbols, which bonded us into the culture of nursing. Mostly these were acceptable abbreviations and didn't often stray into well-known and at one time, accepted medical slang. (see box p. 33)

We folded in the sides of our starched white aprons when sitting for report to keep the front clean, or alternatively cover up anything that might have soiled the front. Some scribbled notes on these inside flaps, or even on the inside of the pinafore at the top. Others grabbed paper towels or paper used for writing patient notes. These days most wards have a printed handover sheet and rules about putting it in the confidential box for shredding before leaving the ward to protect any patient identifiable information.

It is more usual now to have a ward handover where everyone is given a flavour of the needs and complexity of all the patients with one senior nurse in charge or 'coordinating'. Each nurse is allotted four to six patients, often more, and receives an individual, detailed handover by the patient's bed from the nurse who was looking after them. The old-fashioned ritual of getting everything done before lunch is often tested at this point with the incoming nurse pointing out everything that has not been done by the nurse handing over, conveniently ignoring the fact that a patient's day lasts all day.

Research has shown that, unsurprisingly, the quality of the handover affects subsequent nursing care – inaccuracies or omission of information may lead to mistakes or an area of care being overlooked. In an era where everyone knew exactly what was to be done for every patient (whether they needed it or not), mistakes of omission were less likely – or maybe there were fewer, less complicated interventions.

Potentially, the ward handover could be a place for support, encouraging 'team building', although I've not witnessed this very often. It is often a relief after a tough shift to hand over responsibility to someone else as you leave work at the door. All too often, insufficient time is allotted to handover and, as no one is paid more if they arrive early or stay late, handover can be rushed.

For Lee, in the 1960s, at the end of a stretch of fourteen nights on a children's orthopaedic ward, handing over to the morning staff was a relief after a long night and a very busy early morning getting all the various jobs done in time. The children were confined to their cots in plaster of Paris, hip spica, gallows traction or heavy leather CDH (congenital dysplasia of hip) flexion/abduction splints. It was 07.00 and

Lee had everything done early. Kardex written and temperature charts in bed-order on sister's desk, rubber draw sheets washed and hanging up on the line.

> Demob happy I started dancing the polka to 'The Teddy Bears Picnic' – round and round the ward I danced taking turns to take a toy from each child to be my dance partner. Shrieks of laughter. Did I get the time wrong or was sister early? There she was, at the ward door looking grim. Sheer terror. I managed to fumble my way through report … sure I would be sent to matron's office. Report over. Sister said: 'Thank you, you may go Nurse Fahey' But then: 'Next time Nurse, perhaps turn the music down a little.'

For many years nursing notes were recorded in what was called the 'Kardex' – similar to index cards but designed to go inside a slim metal holder where it was possible to flick through all the nursing notes for patients on a ward. Nurses would summarise the patient's care and status in a brief paragraph at the end of each shift. It varied from ward to ward how much detail you included, whether notes were written in the Kardex or in the patient's notes alongside the doctor's notes, or whether there was an entirely different system altogether. Invariably medical and surgical wards would take a different approach which was confusing.

Again, we were not taught the all-important skill of how to record the nursing care given. The emphasis was on learning practical skills. There were a series of stock phrases that nurses tended to employ, particularly when on nights when either nothing had happened, or so much had happened that apart from the complete commotion surrounding a couple of patients, the night staff couldn't remember how the rest of the ward had fared.

These stock phrases included: 'slept well', 'good night's sleep,' and 'no complaints of pain' (did anyone ask?). Diana worked at the RIE in the late 1960s and remembers one sister who did away with the ritual reporting of a patient's condition at the end of a shift. Instead, she wrote the Kardex up first thing in the morning saying what care the patient needed that day and other comments were only written in the Kardex if they were significant. Diana says: 'Woe betide you if you wrote "patient slept well", because she would chat to said patient and discover that they had a horrible night.'

Alison attended a National Association of Theatre Nurses conference in the US in the 1970s where she learned the mantra: 'What isn't written down – wasn't done'. The American experience with litigation emphasising this.

> I realised that we had high standards of patient care in the operating theatre – but were not recording this adequately enough to prove what had taken place. We just 'did it!' So although we all hate paper work, we ensured that we recorded more than we had previously.

Medical slang

Medical slang and/or the use of acronyms is a time honoured method of communication among hospital staff. Generally, the acronyms look impressive and give a visual code that is effective but bordering on the unethical and may refer rudely to something quite unmedical about the patient. Some argue that they accurately and speedily describe a situation and provide some light relief in stressful circumstances. While they can serve as verbal shorthand, most are banned from hospital notes not least because the acronym could refer to a true medical condition and the patient could be incorrectly treated.

Acopia   Description of anyone, from harassed junior doctor to a frail patient unable to live at home unaided.

Ash Cash   System in the UK where junior doctor is paid for signing a cremation form.

Bagging   Manually helping a patient breathe usually during a cardiac arrest using a bag valve mask known as an Ambu Bag which covers mouth and nose.

B/P   Blood pressure;

Code Brown A faecal incontinence emergency. Often used by nurses and medical technicians in theatre requesting help cleaning up an unexpected bowel movement.

EETH   Tried everything else, try homeopathy

ETOH	Alcohol intoxication
Fat Fair Forty & Female	Gall bladder problems common in women who look like this.
FLK	Funny Looking Kid
FLKJLD	Funny Looking Kid Just Like Dad
GWPR	Guardian Women's Page Reader
Handbag positive	Confused patient (usually elderly lady) lying on hospital bed clutching handbag.
Hasselhoff	A term for when a patient presents with an injury for which there is a bizarre explanation. The source is Baywatch actor David Hasselhoff, who hit his head on a chandelier while shaving. The broken glass severed four tendons and an artery in his right arm.
NFA	No Fixed Abode (someone who is homeless)
NFTW	Normal for Tunbridge Wells or wherever patient is from.
O-sign	A patient is very sick, 'giving the O-sign', lying with his mouth open. This is followed by:
Q-sign	When the tongue hangs out of the mouth – when the patient becomes terminal.
PFO	Pissed, fell over.
POP	Plaster of Paris.
SOB	Shortness of breath.
TAH	Total Abdominal Hysterectomy.
TMG	Too Much Grog.
UBI	Unexplained Beer Injury.
UTI	Urinary tract infection.

Chapter 4

Hygiene and Hijinks

'The test of a capable nurse is a patient who feels the better for his blanket bath – relaxed but not worn out with over-exertion; warm but not overheated.'

Traditionally, hospital patients start the day with an early morning wash – sometimes very early. Beleaguered night staff stumbled about in the dark getting patients washed and the ward immaculate before the morning staff arrived. It was a tall order and some nurses employed quite unorthodox tactics to kick off early ablutions.

In the 1950s, Eileen worked on a large chest-ward caring for lung cancer and tuberculosis (TB) patients and remembers that very occasionally the ward cat, Pussy Darling (kept to control the mice population), was fed a quarter tablet of Dexedrine at about 04.00 which would make it race about the ward creating a commotion and waking up some of the patients, the sickest of whom were then given an early wash and bed change to alleviate the morning rush. The cat, apparently unharmed, was rewarded with saucers of cream meant for the TB patients.

One night Pussy Darling suffered a different fate. She escaped. The nurses spent much of the night calling her back in. Eventually, the cat returned and, fearful she would escape again, a nurse popped her in the kitchen plate warmer to keep her safe and cosy until morning. Unfortunately, when she opened the door Pussy Darling was more than a little drowsy. A quick consultation with colleagues and the nurse raided the drugs trolley for some whisky and splashed some in Pussy Darling's face to wake her up. With all the drugs and alcohol, it's a wonder Pussy Darling survived her time on the wards.

However, she got her own back. One night she chased a mouse up the trouser leg of a doctor who was kneeling by a bed aspirating a patient's lung. Eileen says: 'He managed to keep the needle in.'

The problem with working in the dark is that you can't always see what you are doing. Jacqui recalls coming on duty one morning and seeing all the patients sitting up in bed washed and wearing shrouds.

Usually, patient washes take place after morning handover from night staff to day staff. Senior nurses get on with the drug round, while health care assistants (and in previous generations, student nurses) get on with the washes. For many decades, the routine of washing patients changing beds and making sure the ward was clean and tidy felt like an overriding focus of the nursing role – but that might just be how I remember it.

There is an important caring aspect to that morning ritual of washing – one that some claim registered nurses miss out on these days because it is done by HCAs. The opportunity for more social and emotional interaction with the patient and the chance to observe their general condition, their skin, their mobility and their mood. It was a good way to build a rapport with patients and observe them without appearing to be directly checking on them.

According to Wolf in *Rituals of Nursing* (2016), washing and tidying is how nurses impose a sense of order. There is no doubt that order creates confidence that all is under control and that patients are well cared for. In the early 1920s, when nursing had little to offer other than compassion, kindness and cleanliness, warm baths were touted as 'one of the most valuable forms of treatment', and bed bathing was considered an invaluable skill: 'Simple cleanliness of the skin conduces greatly to a patient's feeling of well-being'. (*Groves, Brickdale & Nixon's Text-book for Nurses* 1940s)

Wolf refers to a number of more modern nursing texts which claim that bathing and good hygiene help patients feel better. Warm baths help to relax muscles and ease pain.

For Florence Nightingale, of course, cleanliness of the nurse, the patient and the patient's bed and environment were essential for improving health. She believed it was vital to keep the pores of the skin 'free from all obstructing excretions' (or the patient would be) 'poisoned via the skin as surely as if they had ingested poison'.

In *Notes on Nursing,* Florence writes: 'Every nurse ought to be careful to wash her hands very frequently during the day. If her face too, so much the better.'

While those thinking of nurse training at the RIE, circa 1930s, were advised by one Miss Gill that nurses would have to wash their hair more frequently than at home – at least every two weeks. She also advised that there was a right way and a wrong way to do any task and nurses needed to train themselves to do things the right way. Years spent 'muddling through' was of no use to anyone.

While these days face and hair washing is assumed, hand hygiene is ingrained in everyone's psyche. Wards conduct hand-washing audits to check that everyone is washing their hands properly and at the appropriate moments. Visitors to the wards are invited to clean their hands with sanitiser gel at the entrance.

In the RCN oral history collection, Mary Brown remembers that all new patients had to have their hair washed and a solution applied if nits were discovered; the nurse would then tie a white triangular bandage over the patient's hair – presumably to identify any stray nits or perhaps, mortifyingly, to alert everyone else to their status.

Eileen remembers the standard admission procedure for new patients when she was nursing at a hospital in Kent in the 1950s and recorded in the admissions book:

> Hair. Tooth comb if necessary
> Teeth: Check dentures
> Ears: Must be clean
> Temperature, pulse, respirations (TPR): Check
> Umbilicus: Must be clean
> Weight: Check
> Pre-op: Dettol bath

Various hygiene tasks were allocated to any student who looked vaguely idle. Tracy remembers doing a denture round; having a bowl of water on a trolley as she pushed it around the ward, washing people's false teeth in it. She says while she hoped she changed the water, she doesn't remember doing so.

Jacqui, throwing all the dentures into a sink of water to scrub, didn't think about each patient's dentures being bespoke to them. Too late, she realised that sorting out which set belonged to which patient was impossible. My aunt Molly, aged 90, remembers a friend she trained alongside doing the same thing, forty years earlier. Evidence perhaps of how ritual can overtake thought.

Equipment these days is high tech, often protected by disposable covers and cleaning is done using paper towels and water. In the 1980s old fashioned mercury thermometers were still being used. These were stowed in a little test tube on the wall by each patient's bed. Imagine the horror of the student nurse who on her second day was told to clean the thermometers and busily washed them in hot water, breaking them all.

It's not clear how thermometers were cleaned in one hospital in the Netherlands where Diana worked in the 1970s. A nurse would go around handing out thermometers to patients. Each thermometer was covered in a plastic bag. All patients who were able to would insert the thermometer into their rectums. The nurse would then collect in the thermometers. But some patients got fed up waiting and would take them out and perch them on their lockers – often on the edge of a saucer.

As Ann noted in her studies in 1933 at the Royal Infirmary Edinburgh, cleanliness is the keystone of health and that personal hygiene includes internal cleanliness as well. By this she meant that there was adequate ventilation in the room that the patient's lungs were free of catarrh, their muscles in good condition so they could lie comfortably with their limbs aligned.

The importance of fresh air and the removal of effluvia (an unpleasant or harmful odour or discharge) was a strong belief in Florence Nightingale's time and still lingered through the twentieth century. It was a part of sanitarianism – which aimed to reduce environmental pollution in the interests of human health – and was a theory that preceded germ theory. Indeed, it is still promulgated by those who think we may be over zealous in sterilising our homes and risking the inability of our immune systems to deal with regular bacteria.

In his study of *Nursing Practices used in the Management of Infection in Hospitals, 1929–1948*, David Justham reports that nursing practice at this time placed enormous emphasis on cleanliness and hygiene. Probationer nurses were taught to manage infection risks both to themselves and their patients in a disciplined and safe way. This was achieved through the exercise of strict routines and a hierarchy of tasks. It's easy to see therefore how some of the rituals of nursing became so ingrained – they were vital to protecting the health of both nurse and patient.

Tuberculosis

The tuberculosis sanatoria in the early part of the twentieth century were the epitome of this fresh air approach. Patients were wheeled out onto verandas to spend the day, and often the night, outside, regardless of the weather. This was based on the findings of botany student Hermann Brehmer that sunlight can kill the TB bacteria; Brehmer had TB and found respite in the Himalayan mountains. Similar arrangements for sanatoria were established worldwide and this approach continued into the 1950s. The symptoms of TB were treated with tonics, cod-liver oil, malt and good diet.

Tuberculosis can occur in anyone who has been in prolonged contact with someone who is infectious. It is associated with poor living conditions and overcrowding and is common among those who are homeless. It is a complex disease caused by bacteria and is spread by coughing and sneezing and has been around for centuries.

There are different kinds of TB with the most common being pulmonary TB which affects the lungs. In 1882, the scientist Robert Koch identified the micro-organism that caused TB and this led eventually to a vaccine against the disease and to kinder treatments. Until then, apart from fresh air and a good diet, surgery was the standard treatment. Surgery was done to create an artificial pneumothorax by collapsing the lung and inserting air or nitrogen into the pleural space around the lungs. Other surgery included a thoracoplasty, a surgical procedure to remove ribs from the chest wall. The efficacy of these surgical procedures was never fully proved. The advent of antibiotics in the shape of Rifampicin and other anti-TB drugs in the 1960s, radically transformed the prognosis for people.

Once the patient's high temperature had normalised, they were allowed to exercise gently and later to work – within the hospital grounds – interspersed with frequent rest hours. These patients were in hospital for a long time.

Kathleen, who completed a year of fever nursing in a children's hospital in Manchester, says:

> These poor patients had to be in the cold, the wet and the rain. Rickets patients also had to have fresh air. They lived out on the balcony. It was freezing cold. Snow would be on their beds in the morning.

Evelyn, speaking in an interview with the RCN oral history collection, trained in Bridgend between 1947 and 1951. She remembers nursing children with pneumonia out on the balconies all through winter. 'They were absolutely swathed in warm clothing and we used to make little Gamgee jackets for them.... They had little red noses when they were out there.'

It was thought that this was also good treatment for pneumonitis (a non-infectious inflammation of the lungs). 'It was not so good for the night nurses. You didn't put a coat on – you would have been "disciplined" but you had your cape – only a short one to the shoulders!'

Eileen says that even at night in the depths of winter, the nurses could not wear cardigans over their uniforms when they went out to the patients. She says squirrels used to sit on their beds and beg for snacks.

Wildlife in the wards could also be a problem. Diana remembers preparing a tray of glass syringes for injection on a TB ward in the 1960s, extracting them from the steriliser only to have pigeons swoop in through the open windows of the ward and fly over the tray bringing the sterile nature of the syringes into question.

There has been a resurgence of tuberculosis in recent years and an emergence of multidrug-resistant TB often occurring in patients whose immune systems are already compromised, for example, those who have HIV. Surgery is again part of the armoury for these patients, often for diagnostic purposes using mini-invasive techniques compared to the major surgery of the first half of the twentieth century.

Bed baths

Giving a bed bath is still one of the first procedures any student nurse will perform. First the curtains were pulled around the bed and after careful explanation of what was planned – patients weren't generally given a choice – their top bedclothes were stripped, folded back in thirds away to the foot of the bed keeping them suitably covered with a sheet that could be adjusted as the wash proceeded, and a towel used to maintain the patient's modesty. Next step was to fill a bowl with warm water, test the temperature with your elbow and carry the bowl on a tray to the bedside, with the water perilously close to spilling.

The order of the wash was: front first – face, neck, right arm, torso, left arm, back, if the patient was able to sit up. Cover the patient up to keep warm. Wash the groin. Change the water. Left leg, right leg, 'log roll' the patient to clean back and bottom. We were taught to pat the skin dry and not rub it as this was kinder, especially for delicate skin. Towels or blankets were strategically placed to ensure patients were kept warm and not exposed. We were taught that bed baths always required two towels for drying 'top and tail'.

Routine kept us focused on the process and we were not expected to question it. Some made the mistake of thinking that no one took the bed bath ritual too seriously and one nurse went so far as to question it. The dressing down she received from her clinical tutor left her reeling and she says: 'I have never strayed from the "Bart's way" of washing a patient in bed again.'

Alison says she sat, wide-eyed and rigid with terror at handover on her first shift on her second ward. It had come to the attention of the junior sister, that some nurses had been blanket bathing their patients without stripping the bed correctly first. The sister delivered a devastating broadside to all who sat there about the inappropriateness of this practice and that it was to stop, now. The new recruits held their breath, as she turned to them and kindly excused them from the ticking-off as she knew they were not guilty. They breathed again but ensured they were never guilty of the crime of incorrect preparations of the bedclothes for a bed bath.

My aunt Molly who trained in the 1940s dared to question the strict ritual of 'how things must be done'. She was bathing a patient who was sitting on a rubber ring – used to relieve pressure on the posterior. Molly saw fit to leave the patient on the ring until the first part of the wash was done only removing it when she moved him on to his side. The sister was most displeased telling her the ring had to be removed at the start of the wash because that was the order of things – clearly a better reason than the patient's comfort.

Another of aunt Molly's patients was a wealthy jockey whose stubbornness was legendary. He claimed his family were only interested in him now he was near the end of his life and hoped to benefit from his money, so he refused to see them. Molly was directed to give him a bed bath but was unable to persuade him to remove his all-in-one long johns. Uneasily, she assisted him with washing what was not covered – his hands, face and feet – and prayed sister would not pop her head round the curtains to check. On reflection she realised that sister would have already known of the man's predilection of refusing to remove his underclothes so lived in trepidation of being asked how the bed bath had gone.

Such a strict routine was helpful to those of us who were not yet blasé at the sight of a stranger's naked body. On my first ward – male medical – there seemed to be an awful lot of bed baths and when I look back, I'm quite sure most of those men were capable of washing themselves and I wonder if half the time we 'first warders' were directed to do bed baths to improve our skills and keep us busy (the days of wards being well staffed).

I quickly became wise to when someone was well enough to wash themselves and I would hand them a cloth and the instruction to wash themselves and meekly they would. Occasionally you would be caught out and realise someone was pretending to be helpless: they would give a sly laugh when they realised you had guessed.

Georgina recounts how she assisted one elderly man to wash himself independently by the bedside, helped him dress and return to bed. As she turned to leave, he tapped her bottom as he said thank you. The next day, Georgina got everything ready for the same gentleman.

> He was very smiley ... I left him behind the curtains to wash. Then I heard 'nurse, nurse', I popped my head round the curtain. There he sat holding out a tub of cream with a huge denture free gummy smile saying he wanted me to help him put the cream in reachable places.

When she advised him that if he was capable of tapping her on the bottom yesterday then he was capable of applying his own cream, he replied with a chuckle: 'it was worth a try!'

There were remedies for the uninitiated and unnerved: Mary was in the first intake of nurses to be trained in the new NHS. Her second ward was a male medical ward, where they also carried bowls of warm water to the bedside for bed baths. She says: 'They were mostly young men who were saucy as young men are. They used to ping our suspenders!'

The ward sister had advice for reducing what were described to Mary as any 'tent poles' that might occur during bed baths. Apparently, a dab of surgical spirit applied with some cotton wool soon dampened any young man's ardour.

However, others were delighted to hear of any 'manly responses'. Marina recalls looking after a gentleman who had suffered a severe stroke.

> He had lain paralysed and virtually unconscious for weeks, tube fed and frequently turned to alleviate bed sores. As I bent over him to straighten out the bed sheet, I felt a hand glide up the back of my thigh. I looked around but it was just the two of us, no other person in sight.

Not a little shaken by this, Marina told sister, who exclaimed, beaming from ear to ear: 'Oh good, that's the first sign of his recovery. The sexual urge gets them every time!'

While these incidents might be at the more extreme, there was still considerable learning required to cope with providing intimate care for an almost total stranger. Perhaps this experience contributed to developing the no-nonsense demeanour that is the stereotypical cover for any nurse. A demeanour that can also be something of a cover for rituals themselves – especially those where there is little evidence of their effectiveness, or the evidence for which might be long forgotten.

Sitz baths or salt baths and Savlon baths fall into this category. Sitz baths are still recommended today post-operatively or for women post-childbirth – sitz baths are in fact a shallow bath of warm water just deep enough to sit in. From the German 'sitzen', meaning to sit, they were thought to be soothing after gynaecological or bowel surgery. The premise is that salt added to the water creates a saline solution, helping to keep a wound clean. Over the years, the word sitz has tended to be used interchangeably with salt, although one has to question just how much salt is needed if it is to be worthwhile. Gail, who trained in the late 1970s, says:

> In PTS (preliminary training school) we were taught how to calculate the amount of salt to add to a bath to make a 0.9% saline solution. Imagine our surprise when we got on the wards and found that you just threw a cupful in – no calculation or weighing required!

A study in a large general hospital by Austin in the 1980s found that twenty-six wards out thirty-five used salt baths for all manner of conditions from rashes to pressure sores but of course the depth of the water and the quantity of salt varied from nurse to nurse, never mind ward to ward, so actualising the exact therapeutic amount (if there ever was one) was impossible. Research published in 1988 by Sleep and Grant found no significant difference in wound healing between three different groups: those who added a 100ml sachet of Savlon to a post-operative bath, those who added salt or those who stuck with plain water.

Mustard baths, according to *Modern Professional Nursing*, were thought ideal for tired bodies, colds, fevers and seizures. The mustard, in the form of mustard seeds, added to a very hot bath, was thought to draw out toxins and warm the muscles, blood and body.

In later years, we came to realise that those bowls of water, rinsed and stored behind the patient's locker and used for their daily washes, might be a source of infection and should have had a more rigorous deep clean than the rinse and spray we gave them with Sudol solution. Sudol, had its own problems because it was kept in a refillable bottle but the bottles were never themselves cleaned and quite likely harboured bacteria.

As the realities of hospital-acquired infections began to creep in, the days of these bowls and bottles came to an end and disposable cardboard bowls became the norm. However, these are not strong enough to hold much water and so post-operative patients very often have to make it to the bathroom, however lousy they feel. While probably good for their mobilisation, there just seems a mild lack of compassion in this approach, but it is all about getting the patient home as quickly as possible.

Arguably, the health service is not there to provide anything other than healthcare, but at one time a tiny tablet of soap, toothbrush and toothpaste were provided for the very many patients who didn't own such things or came into hospital as an emergency.

Some departments even had washing machines and nurses would do the laundry for patients. One remembers:

> I loved being able to wash patient's clothing, especially when they didn't have relatives to help. I think the strangest thing I was asked to wash was a sleeping bag (my patient was homeless). It took 5 washes to get it totally clean, but he was so chuffed with it.

Hygiene for those who are homeless and often living on the streets can be quite impossible and they are at risk of a range of health conditions exacerbated by their living arrangements – anything from coughs and colds to skin disease, even tuberculosis. They often seek a safe haven at night in a corner of A&E. At one time referred to in patient's notes, as NFAs (no fixed abode), sometimes they wander in on their own or are brought in by the police or by ambulance if they are injured or very inebriated. Rosie says: 'In A&E you know your regulars; you know which ones you can let in the waiting room and give them a tea and a cheese sandwich.'

Others, who might be trouble, are encouraged to move on. Rosie remembers one regular, Bill, who had asthma and when his chest was bad, he could come into A&E: 'We kept a Ventolin inhaler with his name on at the nurses' station and we would give him a couple of puffs and make him a cup of tea and send him on his way.'

One Sunday, when Bill came in looking particularly unkempt and smelling worse, the A&E sister beckoned Rosie over and the two of them took him to the huge bathrooms that were underground, beneath the outpatients' department. 'Never expect your staff to do something you wouldn't do yourself,' was one of this sister's mantras. So together, she and Rosie donned gloves, aprons and masks and gently stripped off Bill's maggot- and lice-ridden clothes and put him in the bath, shaving his head and trimming his nails. Every A&E has a stock of spare clean clothes, so Bill was provided with these, while his old clothes were binned. Rosie says: 'You would not have the time nowadays, and you probably wouldn't be allowed to do all that.'

Sometimes, rules are there to be bent a little to give care to someone who needs it, she says.

Mary Anne recalls from her days in A&E that when homeless people came in needing care and attention, their clothes, more often than not, had to be cut off as they were so badly caked in faeces and running with maggots and fleas.

> We used fairly high force showers on these poor people, while trying to keep dry ourselves. It was not a job we enjoyed. I once begged not to have to clean one person, as I saw a large black spider disappear up his trouser leg!

Jackie remembers spiders floating to the surface of the bath water as she helped homeless visitors to get clean, often trimming their beards and cutting their hair too, all part of the ritual of making them 'presentable' and ensuring they could be examined. Just like eating and drinking, feeling clean is the one definite improvement you can offer someone who spends their life on the street. 1940s *Modern Professional Nursing* declares: 'Even the tramp knows that he feels a better man after his hot bath: the moral effect is of great tonic value; indeed, if he had it more often he would not be a tramp.'

While it seems a tall order for regular baths to rescue you morally and physically from street life, there is no doubt that washing is one of the first caring steps that are offered, not only to help someone feel better but also to identify any underlying health problems.

Chapter 5

Egg White and Oxygen

'I'll have a B cup like you nurse.'

It is not clear when egg white and oxygen made an appearance but universally, twentieth-century nurses in the UK will know it as *the* treatment for pressure sores. It involved smearing egg white onto an open bed sore and then drying it with high flow oxygen via a mask attached to the oxygen supply at the wall. How this came to be an acceptable treatment is unclear. According to David Barton, now retired associate professor of nursing: 'Egg white is protein, and oxygen is good for cells, so it made some sense.'

However, he adds: 'we know now that eggs can be infected with salmonella and there is a fair bit of evidence that their use in pressure ulcer therapy was fairly catastrophic.'

Sugar and raw eggs were another recipe for bedsores. The sugar does have some scientific basis for healing wounds: through osmosis it promotes granulation of healthy tissues and reduces oedema.

Eggs aside, Carol trained in the early 1970s and remembers that although the incidence of bed sores was quite infrequent, there were some weird and wonderful remedies, one of which was to spray insulin onto the sore and use oxygen to dry it. Carol was asked to attend to a gentleman's bed sore and duly sprayed 100-unit strength insulin onto the wound.

> I must have been rather liberal with the insulin (which was not prescribed as the patient was not a diabetic) but I followed sister's dictats. After about 30 minutes the patient did not look very well; indeed, he was slowly slipping into a coma – a hypoglycaemic attack. Boy, was I scared but a

glass of sugared Lucozade duly saved him. Thereafter that treatment was discontinued – on our ward at least – only to be replaced by good old egg white and oxygen!

Also known as black sloughs, trophic ulcers, necrotic ulcers, ischaemic ulcers, decubitus ulcers, pressure ulcers or sores are localised damage to the skin and/or the underlying tissue and occur when there is pressure on an area caused by lying or sitting on it and constricting the blood flow, usually over a bony prominence on the body. The lower back, the heels and tips of the shoulders as well as the back of the head and the elbows are all at risk.

Recorded as far back as ancient Egypt, arguments as to their cause and, more pertinently, who is to 'blame' for them have been around for ever. In the nineteenth century, the physician Jean-Martin Charcot (who first described multiple sclerosis and whose name is linked to a number of conditions) believed that pressure sores or ulcers were an unavoidable result of damage to the brain or spinal cord.

This theory was challenged by another French physician, Henri Brown-Sequard who believed, correctly as it turned out, that it was compression on an area and not lack of nerve supply that led to pressure sores. However, the nerve damage theory persisted until as recently as the 1940s, which meant that the medical profession was sceptical about the chances of preventing and treating the ulcers and left care of pressure sores to nurses.

As a result, they have long been considered evidence of poor nursing – from Margaret Broadley's time in the 1920s, to my mother's in the 1950s, to mine in the 1980s. As Carol says: 'We were ashamed as a ward if a patient got a bed sore.'

They most commonly develop in people who are immobile. Shearing the skin can lead to sores developing. Woe betide those nurses who, in the days when it was acceptable to lift patients, failed to lift them fully and dragged them up the bed instead, causing skin damage.

Prevention is the key, because once pressure sores develop, they are, as the weird remedies are testament to, very difficult to treat, especially in critically ill people who may suffer from incontinence or whose nutrition may be poor. Wet skin breaks down very quickly. Some conditions such as paralysis or neuropathy (nerve damage) reduce sensation in the skin and contribute to the risk of sores developing.

Whatever their generation, nurses have known that the only way to prevent pressure sores was to ensure patients didn't lie or sit in one spot for too long. But even the two-hour window we allowed ourselves between moving or turning patients who were bed-bound was not always enough to stop them. I'm not convinced that the two hours was based on scientific evidence. More than likely it fitted ward routine and the frequency with which patients could tolerate being disturbed.

As well as moving patients, all kinds of powder or potions were applied to skin that was in danger of breaking down, often causing more damage than it prevented. The routine of back care began as far back as the early twentieth century and was known as the 'back round'. Ida started her training at the Royal Infirmary Edinburgh (RIE) in 1918. In her account with the RCN oral history collection, she says:

> First day I went to the nurse's home at 6pm and I was on the ward at 7pm... I was helping with a patient not a day or two afterwards and the nurse said to me 'Go and get the back tray'. So, I rushed off to the kitchen and brought out a big black tray [and] put it under the bed ... I caused confusion I can tell you. It was the back tray for doing the backs, you see [that she wanted].

The back tray or trolley remained in existence for another generation or two. In aunt Molly's day in the 1940s and 1950s, the back round was a strict regime, the three essential rules of which were: maintain absolute cleanliness, avoid prolonged pressure and stimulate the circulation of the part.

Cleanliness involved a wash twice a day, or every time the patient was incontinent. After washing, the nurse was supposed to soap her hand well (remember no gloves) and apply the soap to the patient's back and rub until it was absorbed, leaving the skin dry. Next, she tipped methylated spirit into her hand and rubbed it into the skin until it was pink and dry. Lastly, she rubbed in starch powder, paying special attention to the fold of the buttocks. Sometimes zinc and castor oil ointment or boracic ointment was used instead of the methylated spirit. Molly doesn't say what this variety of potions did to her hands, never mind the patients' skin.

Arachis (peanut) oil and methylated spirit was another remedy applied vigorously to patients across Glasgow, often to paper thin sacral areas with the justification that the oil softened the skin and the meths toughened it, as if that was a solution.

Doreen says she and her colleagues carried out a back round three or four times a day, which meant straightening sheets and rubbing backs and heels. Looking back, she says it was not always necessary but it was a good way of spending time with patients and getting to know them, while also being busy, which was vital.

Michael echoes this, saying that the back round on his first ward – a male orthopaedic ward in the 1960s – was important not only for the prevention of pressure sores among those bed-bound in traction, but also for getting to know the patients. Learning to talk with them and to listen.

The use of apparatus to apply traction to injured limbs has been part of the treatment of patients with fractures since the time of the Ancient Greeks. It is used less and less these days as the combination of innovative surgical treatment and antibiotics and a more active approach to rehabilitation, means that bone fractures can be pinned and plated and patients mobilised and discharged quite quickly. However, traction does still have its place and good nursing care is required to make sure the traction is well maintained and patient's pressure areas well attended to.

Jacqui's second ward in the 1980s was male orthopaedic. Traction was still very much in use but the patients were often young men with limb fractures following bike accidents or footballing injuries.

Apart from the broken limb, they were generally quite fit and not a little bored. Jacqui says, she and her fellow students were very naïve, giving them all bed baths. One young man was in a hip to toe plaster, and the only instruction Jacqui had been given in a throw-away line from the staff nurse was to make sure that because he was in plaster nothing was swollen. It was not explained to Jacqui, but swelling under the plaster cast could be the first indication of a serious condition which would necessitate immediate removal of the plaster to reduce pressure. Jacqui says:

> So, I go to see him and pull the curtains round and he whips off the sheet to show his impressive erection. I screamed put the sheet back over him rushed to the office, grabbed the resus box, for some reason, exclaiming 'it's swollen, it's

swollen you better come and look'. The sister and the staff nurse came thundering after me: this poor guy with this impressive thing certainly deflated fast enough.

Jacqui says: 'I think that's when I was sent to theatre to ask for a long stand. So, I did. Forty five minutes later I twigged that a long stand was not a piece of apparatus, it was a long stand.'

There are associated delicate areas of the body that are susceptible to skin damage and soreness from lying in bed. Cate says she worked with one ward sister who was obsessed with elevating scrotums at night onto foam pads. There did not seem to be any medical reason for this and the same practice was applied to all the male patients. Cate says: 'It was a hoot. I think this was actually outlawed practice that was continued by one particular ward sister who had been indoctrinated in training.'

Scrotal support was important for men post hernia operations, but how much support was offered by the handknitted items made by the good ladies of the Women's Royal Voluntary Service (WRVS) is unclear; more sweaty and itchy than supportive. They came in three sizes which the nurse was required to hold up in front of the patient for him to choose an appropriate size. Not many requested a 'small' – referred to as a Brussels sprout holder, while it wasn't uncommon for a patient to reply: 'I'll have a B cup like you nurse.'

One student remembers a senior nurse telling her that the way you could tell which size you required for the patient was by cupping your hands around the patient's testicles and allowing them to fall naturally. 'She said that as I had large hands if they fitted snuggly it would be large. It was a moment before I realised she was joking.'

Anne-Marie was flummoxed by how to fit the support for one older gentleman as gravity had taken its toll. 'My advice ever since to former boyfriends, husband and my boys is to wear boxers with support not those old fashioned loose ones!'

Other items to offer comfort and prevention of sores included sheepskin fleeces, similar to numnahs worn under saddles when horse riding. These were soft and gentle on the skin but were also very warm and caused patients to sweat while not really relieving pressure. Rubber rings covered with a pillow case and popped onto the unforgiving ward chairs relieved pressure in one area but tended to create it in another. In the 1980s these cushions came readymade but in the 1940s, they had to be blown up. Nurses were cautioned to always use a pump and not: 'Commit the outrage against asepsis by blowing up the bag with their own breath.' (*Modern Professional Nursing Vol II.*)

Bed cradles, a frame placed under the bedclothes effectively lifted the weight of them off the patient. Monkey poles – in place over the bed so patients could heave themselves up – were all well and good for strong patients who could lift themselves without dragging on the bed but of no use to the weak and frail, who were in danger of dislocating a shoulder.

Still pressure sores occurred and unusual remedies continued. A report in 1990 found that nurses tended to carry out what it called the 'time honoured practice' of treating them with Edinburgh Solution of Lime (Eusol). It certainly cleaned up the ulcers creating the impression of effective treatment. However, Eusol was later found to be a skin irritant that destroyed healthy tissue, slowing wound healing. It was also a likely cause of cancer. Its use was eventually withdrawn.

Diana worked at a hospital near Rotterdam in the Netherlands in the late 1970s where patients were never turned. Pressure sores were treated with ice cubes rubbed round the edge of the open sore followed by a warm blast from a hair dryer. The combination of making the open sores wet and cold and then hot and dry makes no sense and Diana says she never noticed any improvement.

Martin trained as a mental health nurse. He says:

> In the Victorian asylum where I trained in the late 1960s, early 1970s, there were 'sick' wards for the physically frail and unwell. As a second year student on my first day on the sick ward I accompanied the sister on her treatment rounds for these sores, some of which were open, gaping wounds, the sight of which could turn even the strongest stomach.

The sister prepared a trolley of sterile dressing packs, gauze swabs, tape, forceps and also a large jar of Marmite.

> Sadly, and almost unbelievably, once sister had removed old dressings and cleaned the wounds, she then packed them with the Marmite. In ignorance, I assumed this was routine treatment, researched, validated and approved. Only later

did I learn that this was a very personal idiosyncrasy of that sister who believed that the protein in the Marmite would stimulate tissue growth.

This practice went unchallenged and it was only when the sister retired that Martin overheard others laughing about her obsession.

Worse than this sort of ignorance were those who knew that turning patients was important but refused to do it. Seconded to a local hospital as part of my training, I worked with the established night staff. They refused point blank to move from the nurses' station all night, apart from sleeping in the linen cupboard on their break. In the hour before dawn they would tidy up the ward and change beds where patients had been lying in urine waiting for help. This was my introduction to the art of appearing to have done your job when really only the surface has been wiped. You never forget it and can always spot it.

Upsetting the night staff by trying to do the turning on your own was a calculated risk as you had to spend seven nights in their company. Anyway, it is impossible to move another adult on your own without risking shearing their skin or damaging your back. I did report my concerns to the night sister on her rounds and she apologised and acknowledged the situation. She was as helpless as I was. The night staff had been there for years and did not appear to be answerable to anyone.

There were of course those patients – and they were few and far between – who as a result of their own anxiety and fear saw it as their job to make our lives as miserable as possible. In school, we were told that there was no such thing as a difficult patient – a mantra we repeated to each other – often tongue in cheek after a bad day. One nurse on nights who had been treated to all kinds of misery by a particular patient, was stunned when the ward doors flew open in the small hours and a team of nurses (the student's best friend among them) rushed in, pulled the curtains around the bed of the 'difficult patient' and announced that they were the 'pressure area care flying squad' and it was their job to make sure she was washed and turned. They proceeded to give her a full blanket bath and bed change before disappearing into the night. The next morning the patient thought she had dreamt it all and was not at all perturbed. It felt like karma, but it's not clear whether the special treatment had any effect on her demeanour!

Prevention and treatment of pressure sores continued to be ritualistic and haphazard at least until the late 1980s when City and Hackney Health

Authority's Chief Nursing Officer, Pam Hibbs carried out a pioneering ten-year study in East London which did much to transform our understanding and the nursing care of pressure sores. Susie was involved in the project. 'Miss Hibbs was determined that nursing practice should be evidence led, and more importantly designed and done by nurses,'

Pam Hibbs had recognised that there was a very high rate of pressure sores in patients who had a fractured neck of femur, and the received wisdom was that it was due to insufficient care on the wards. Susie's role was to follow every patient admitted to Bart's and the Hackney hospitals with a fractured neck of femur. She monitored all that happened to them including what they were lying on – bed, trolley or theatre table and how long for, examining them for pressure sores every day.

> We found that it was the time they spent on trolleys in A&E and on the theatre table that caused the pressure sores. This led to changes in procedures in A&E to ensure patients were triaged, X-rayed and diagnosed much more quickly, and to pressure relieving mattresses being used in A&E and in theatre.

These days there is talk of avoidable and unavoidable pressure ulcers – no such talk would have been tolerated a generation ago. Then all pressure ulcers were considered avoidable. However, various methods of assessing the patient's risk of developing a pressure sore have come to the fore over the years. One of the most well-known was the Waterlow Score Chart devised in 1985 by Judith Waterlow, who developed it as a comprehensive way for nurses to assess a patient on their admission and reach a 'score' of pressure sore risk.

The scorecard required quite detailed information and too often nurses in their busyness might take a guess at some of the answers in order to reach a conclusion, thus rather negating the final score.

Currently, a simple SKINS system is in place in many hospitals which stands for:

Skin Inspection
Keep moving
Incontinence management
Nutrition and hydration
Surface (on which someone is sitting or lying)

Pressure sores are graded in order to monitor them and to ensure appropriate action is taken. Initially, they may be described superficial – grade 1 – where the skin is red and may be a little warm and doesn't blanche when you press it. Stages 2, 3, 4 and worse follow on.

Lifting and handling

Lifting patients to a better sitting position in bed – the Australian lift – or lifting patients from bed to chair – the cradle or chair lift – was all part of the manual handling that was taught for most of the twentieth century. Student nurses spent many hours in the clinical classroom practising lifting each other. Inevitably it was much easier to lift an average sized 18-year-old girl than later lifting a 20-stone confused patient on a ward, trying not to knock over flowers on the locker or drag the curtains open.

The Australian lift involved a nurse stooping each side of the patient nestling their shoulder into the patient's armpit and together hoiking them up the bed. It could effectively move the patient into a sitting position but may well have harmed their skin if they were inadvertently dragged on the sheet, not to mention risking injury to nurses' backs, and patient's armpits and shoulders.

The cradle lift involved two nurses one either side of the patient sitting in bed or chair, forming a 'cradle by linking hands under the patient's shoulders and then linking hands under the patient's buttocks and lifting together without jerking them.

Studies have since shown that this sort of patient handling was extremely hazardous with substantial risk of causing low back pain or even injury to the people lifting. The risk was even greater for those who lifted on their own, which we were told never to do but invariably you found yourself risking it. This might involve lifting a patient from a seated position on the side of the bed and into a chair. The twisting motion involved was a big part of the risk, never mind the weight of the patient and the danger that they might panic and move suddenly, jarring themselves and the nurse, or even slip to the floor with the nurse trying to 'catch' them.

Studies from that era found that 40,000 nurses reported back-related injuries annually (Garrett et al., 1992). At one time, back injuries in hospital nurses accounted for greater than half the total compensation payments for back injury and it is estimated that more than 764,000 lost work-days were incurred each year.

These days, there is a variety of equipment and aids available including hoists which can be used to lift patients, although this can be a time-consuming and labour-intensive process which usually requires two people to help get the patient safely into and out of a hoist. Staff shortages means this can result in patients waiting a long time to be moved, their wash to be completed and their bed changed.

Chapter 6

Bladders, Bowels and Bodily Functions

'High, hot and a helluva lot!'

Etched on Mary Anne's memory is the bewhiskered, confused gentleman who grabbed his sputum pot as she reached out to take it from his locker and started drinking from it, sputum trailing down from his mouth and into his beard.

Most nurses are squeamish about something – it may be vomit or pus or blood. I remember a staff nurse asking me to look after a patient having a fairly innocuous nose bleed as she couldn't handle them. But everyone recoils at sputum. Sputum is the final frontier. Linda recalls that,

> Emptying and cleaning sputum mugs was the worst job in the world. Gagging, and eyes watering you emptied and scraped the thick sticky phlegm from the stainless-steel container, which you then washed in soapy water and placed in the steriliser.

On her very first day on the isolation ward in 1943, Ruby had to collect up the sputum mugs, dispose of the contents and boil up the mugs in a kettle for 20 minutes to clean them.

Sputum mugs gave way to little plastic sputum pots which at least didn't need washing and could be disposed of once the contents had been inspected. Jan says that as a first warder, her job was to line up the sputum pots on a ledge in the sluice every morning at 07.30, patient's name against each and, with the ward sister breathing down her neck, she would have to describe the contents of each pot.

Lurid descriptions of sputum (and other emissions from the body) used to be common. In her nursing notes of 1932 at the Royal Infirmary Edinburgh, Ann Lamb reports needing to be aware of red currant jelly sputum likely to be due to sarcoma (cancer) of the lung; and black sputum seen in the lungs of miners due to inhalation of coal dust – a condition known as anthracosis – a lung disease that took ten or twenty years to develop.

There were similarly striking descriptions of the patients who had these conditions. 'Blue Bloaters' and 'Pink Puffers' suffered from severe chronic obstructive pulmonary disease (COPD). Blue bloaters had what is now described as chronic bronchitis. They were generally short of breath, causing them to become cyanosed or blue and were often overweight with puffy ankles (bloating). Pink Puffers on the other hand tended to be thin and breathed very fast as they tried to get oxygen to the tissues, so their skin was pink. It's an old term for what we would now describe as severe emphysema. They may also have had what was described as a 'barrel' chest – a symptom of emphysema is not being able to exhale fully so a person's chest might be permanently slightly expanded.

Finger clubbing, commonly seen in smokers, where the tips of the fingers enlarge and the nails curve around the fingertips is another sign of various types of lung disease.

Influenza

Influenza or flu and its secondary infections are the archetypal illnesses for which good nursing care evolved. One hundred years ago the deadliest outbreak of flu was in full swing. The first wave began in 1918, and so-called Spanish flu swept across the globe in waves over the next two years, decimating the lives of mostly young healthy people, often sparing children and the elderly. Knowledge about its cause, its spread, prevention and treatment were all limited.

A report on a conference on influenza in the *British Journal of Nursing* in 1919 shows that doctors were tantalisingly close to understanding the nature and spread of the condition. They considered the possible relation of flu to climate, whether crowding encouraged its spread and whether masks were good protection (still debated in the 2009 H1N1 flu epidemic). The view in 1919 was that the best protection was for the patient to wear the mask (rather than the nurse or doctor); and, while a vaccine against flu was still not available, it was important to protect against secondary bacterial infections. Sir Malcom Morris, President of the Institute of Hygiene chaired the conference. He expressed the opinion that alcohol was not essential, either as a preventive measure or as treatment.

Flu is a viral illness and cannot be cured. Treatment involves caring for its symptoms. Antibiotics are of no value (except for subsequent bacterial infections) but the availability of medicines such as paracetamol to alleviate pyrexia are a vital breakthrough. We encourage the young and the old and those who are vulnerable to respiratory conditions such as asthma to have a flu vaccine each year. The virus mutates from year to year which is why a new vaccine needs to be developed annually.

Healthcare workers such as nurses also protect themselves and those they care for by having the flu vaccine. Recent concern that there are those who have a chronic form of the disease, where they have the condition and can infect others, but don't become ill with it themselves, were raised as long ago as that conference in 1919.

Bowels and bladders

Inevitably, nursing also means poo and pee. As a second-year student I was on a female medical ward at the old Hackney hospital in East London, when a routine bed bath turned into an explosive encounter with a patient's violent diarrhoea. An agency nurse I was working with came to my rescue and as we worked together to clean up the patient, she said to me: 'This is what nursing is all about. Don't let anyone tell you any different.'

I felt disheartened. I really didn't want to be in a job where cleaning up poo was all I could expect. On the upside, I learnt how to hold my breath for quite long periods of time so as not to take in unpleasant smells.

Bowel function is a good barometer of people's health, although I think *Modern Nursing* (1949) exaggerates a little when it describes chronic constipation as a precursor of diseases such as rheumatism, gout and anaemia. However, there is no doubt that questions about bowel habits are something of an obsession in hospitals. When my mother trained as a nurse in the 1950s, the daily question of patients was 'One for the book?' and the answer duly noted in a book recording all patients' bowel activity. There were separate books for weights, routine observations such as temperature, pulse and respiration and for the back round for pressure area care. Some wards maintained this system of books until well into the 1980s.

The bed pan round was a ritual for generations of patients and nurses with bed pans presented to patients after each meal, regardless of whether they wanted one or not. Before the advent of bed pan washers, nurses cleaned the bed pans by hand.

At Manchester Royal Infirmary in the 1960s, two junior nurses were in charge of the bed pan round. Sporting red candy striped gowns over their uniforms. Linda says they first warmed the stainless steel pans under hot water and then stacked them on a large two-shelved trolley. They drew the curtains around the beds and the pans were distributed. After a short interval they were collected and patients assisted with wiping as required. The pans were emptied and put in the pan steriliser. The two nurses then distributed stainless steel bowls filled with warm water from huge jugs so patients could wash their hands. Linda says:

> This was a lengthy process on the female wards and it was always rush, rush, rush. The round on the male ward was much easier, bottles could be carried upright, three to a hand and didn't need warming. Bedpans were needed less often.

Modern Professional Nursing identifies a role for the senior nurse: 'The routine adopted in most hospitals is that the first motion passed by a patient after his admission to a ward is inspected by the sister, or at least by the senior nurse.'

While this is no longer routine, it remains the case that most patients on admission are asked to provide a urine specimen which is checked for signs of infection or other problems. This is worthwhile because urinary tract infections can present in mysterious ways but are easily treatable. Backache might be the first inkling of trouble with your 'waterworks' and, in the elderly, confusion, or increased agitation could be due to a urinary tract infection rather than a sudden onset of dementia. A course of antibiotics and plenty of fluids usually quickly restores people.

In the early 1980s, Mary Anne was working on what were then called the geriatric wards. Patients, especially those with indwelling catheters, were encouraged to drink plenty, especially orange and lemon barley squashes. Mary Anne says: 'These patients often had wee that looked like a brownish pea soup, and smelled worse.'

The hospital took part in research looking at whether drinking cranberry juice had any beneficial effects, so people were asked to volunteer to take part in the study. Within a few days it became overwhelmingly clear that patients who continued to drink the barley cordials had sludgy wee, while those who changed and drank just water were a bit better off but those who drank cranberry juice and water had clear wee within a couple of days.

Urine testing is quick and easy – a simple strip of reagent pads dipped into the urine serves as a diagnostic tool for a range of things such as infection and blood. If the urine is clear with nothing abnormal detected, this is recorded in the patient's notes – very often as NAD – or no abnormalities detected. Although, when I was training there was one ward sister who declared that NAD stood for: Not Actually Done. Nurses were to write out the result in full.

At the Glasgow Royal Infirmary in the 1960s Fay remembers the stink of 'sweetie jars' in the sluice – large glass jars used to store 24-hour urines – collected over this timespan to check in particular for excess protein in the urine. It was the junior nurse's job to take all the jars to a lab room, empty a little urine from each into a glass beaker in order to test it using a urinometer to measure the specific gravity of the urine, then she would lay little squares of blotting paper in front of the jar – one for each test and using different tablets, test for albumen, blood, ketones and sugar. Fay says: 'Early on we boiled the glucose test water but then we got the tablets – 5 drops urine 10 drops water.'

She would then wash all utensils, take the jars back to the sluice to empty and wash them before putting them back on the shelf.

In the 1940s urinalysis was even more complex and mostly had to be done in a laboratory, although there were one or two tests that *Groves and Brickdale* state were so simple that: 'any nurse should be able to perform them accurately'.

In *Sisters* by Barbara Mortimer, Doris Carter, who was a staff nurse at the start of the Second World War, recalls urine testing as being a laborious daily job for the most junior member of the nursing staff: 'You usually spent an hour in the sluice room every morning testing the urines and it wasn't a matter of sticking in a paper, it was all very complicated and every urine had to be tested for everything.'

Care of urinary catheters was often hidebound by ritual. The catheter tube runs from the bladder through the urethra and the risk is that infection can track back up to the sterile bladder and cause an infection. To counter this, nurses would instigate a catheter care regime, referring to the procedure book for the method of care approved by their ward – as likely to be based on the opinion of whoever had written it as any scientific evidence. Careful cleaning around where the tube entered the body – the meatus – was key and an important ritual of the bed bath although I'm not aware of how effective this was at preventing infection rather than introducing it.

Linda worked on a medical ward where a patient had undergone an endoscopy. She says:

> I was told that a camera had been put into the patient's stomach and was lost during the procedure. It was a very expensive piece of equipment and had to be retrieved so the patient was to remain in hospital and we were to collect all of his stools which would be sent to X-ray to try and find the missing camera. To help things along the patient would be given aperients.
>
> The X-ray department had different ideas and after three days of negotiation, they absolutely refused to X-ray excreta. The plastic bags of faeces were piling up in the sluice and the patient was becoming more and more irritated about having to remain in hospital. It was decided that the faeces would be sieved. I was the lucky person chosen for this task and I spent a very unpleasant afternoon with a small meshed kitchen sieve and dessert spoon, pushing faeces through the sieve and searching for the camera. Gloves were not available on the wards in those days. I didn't find the camera and the patient was discharged.

Linda also recalls transporting hot stools from ward to laboratory. She says:

> The stool had to be kept warm and delivered to the laboratory without delay. To achieve this, the patient was given a warmed bedpan and, while he was using it, we filled

a hot water bottle. On receiving the stool, the warm bedpan
was covered with a pan cloth and put on top of the hot water
bottle. The nurse then rushed off to deliver the specimen as
quickly as possible. If the ward was on the first or second
floor the quickest way to the laboratory was via the fire
escape. It was particularly difficult to run down a fire escape
with a bedpan balanced on a hot water bottle, especially in
winter when the steps might be slippery from snow or ice!

Many people fear the embarrassment of having a heart attack during sex,
but truth be told, it's more common to have a heart attack while on the
toilet and certainly more likely in a hospital setting. As an 18-year-old on
my first ward, caring for a man who had been a patient for many weeks,
I was horrified to learn that this was his eventual undignified demise.

Martin, a mental health nurse on secondment to a general ward, was
sent to the toilets to guard against such an event:

> The ward sister explained that one of the potential hazards
> post-heart attack, was that the body shuts down all but
> essential functions during a health emergency, and as
> very few people subsequently feel comfortable perched
> on a bedpan, with nothing but a thin curtain to absorb any
> bodily noises, blocked up bowels were almost inevitable.
> Consequently, whenever such a patient was first able to leave
> their bed – usually a few days after their heart attack – they
> headed straight for the toilet. There, the effort of straining
> to pass a motion could often bring on a second heart attack.

Therefore, Martin was despatched to follow John, four days after
admission, as he ventured on tottery legs to the toilet, to 'make sure he
was okay', although no one explained what Martin was supposed to do
if he wasn't. He says:

> I stationed myself outside his cubicle, ready to rush in,
> should he collapse. I didn't want him to know I was
> eavesdropping so crept around as noiselessly as possible
> while a succession of other patients wandered in and out
> to use the facilities, many of them looking upon me, I felt,

as the sort of pervert who lingers far too long in the public loo in Victoria Station. John was ensconced for rather a long time and of course his strenuous efforts were accompanied by considerable noise and not a little odour. To the relief of us both he didn't bring on a second coronary and as soon as I heard him flush, I scuttled away, lest he should emerge to find me loitering.

It was worse for my friend Liz. Three weeks into her first ward, she realised a patient had died in the toilet and fallen forward with his head pressed against the door so she couldn't open it. A ward round was in progress. Liz crept up to the staff nurse and whispered to her what had happened. On being told to 'just pull the curtains round the bed', Liz explained the patient's whereabouts causing the staff nurse to throw her arms in the air and run off the ward in tears, exclaiming that she couldn't cope. The consultant told his house officer to sort it out and marched off the ward, medical students in tow.

The house officer climbed over the top of the cubicle and moved the patient away from the door and then, says Liz, 'we had to put him in a wheelchair and wheel him through the ward to his bed talking to him as if he were still alive!'

It turned out that the staff nurse's reaction was because her father in Malaysia had died overnight. She asked Liz and another student to carry out last offices, that is, lay out the body. Liz says:

> Neither of us had done it before, so we propped up the procedure book on the locker and did our best. He had already had a wash so we agreed, that with 30 more patients to wash that morning, to not wash him again. We couldn't find a shroud so popped him in a clean hospital gown.

That was Liz's first experience of death.

Alleviating constipation

With hindsight, it could be said that relieving patients of painful bowel conditions or preparing them for bowel surgery was managed in previous decades with a slightly gung-ho approach. *Modern Professional Nursing* speaks of being careful and gentle and, while I like to think that we were, we also thought nothing of pouring water into patients for all manner of reasons.

Alleviating constipation has had many remedies over the years and usually a combination of good diet and keeping hydrated works for those who are fit and well. But once someone is unwell, inactivity and poor diet means everything can grind to a halt.

Croton Oil was one of the more alarming remedies. Known as a cathartic, it was described by *Modern Professional Nursing Vol II* as: 'so powerful, one drop can cause complete watery evacuation … the patient feels as though they have been scrubbed out from within.'

Alice Clegg recorded in her nursing notes of 1924:

> Croton oil is a strong purgative given mostly to unconscious patients. Dose: 1 to 2 minims placed in a small piece of butter to form a pill. Place it far back on the patient's tongue, and it will slide down the throat as it melts.

Placing anything in the throat of an unconscious patient is an alarming thought, particularly when the purpose was to 'scrub them out from within'.

Manual evacuation or disimpaction of the bowel is the ultimate constipation remedy and sometimes necessary for those who have a neurological condition that means they have poor or absent muscle control, such as a spinal injury. Occasionally, other patients also become so impacted that the only remedy is to digitally break up the faeces at the lower end of their bowel. These days, such a procedure is only carried out by a skilled, registered nurse with the explicit consent of the patient. But as Martin recalls of his time working in mental health, it wasn't always so:

> Jim was in his 80s, a small hunched figure with claw like hands and finger nails at least four inches long. His hair and beard were both long and matted. His language was rich, salty, full of aggression and shrieked at ear-splitting volume.

Jim would not let the nursing staff near, him except to help him eat, and would not tolerate anyone touching him, lashing out with his long nails or biting whoever came near. Martin says:

> I had been on Jim's ward less than a week but had already learned to give him a healthy berth when we realised that he was severely constipated. Regrettably, all the usual treatments, both oral and per rectum, failed to produce the desired result so the house officer decided that a manual evacuation was in order.

Martin was assigned this job with the advice and support of four well meaning colleagues. Armed with gloves, lubricant, two bedpans that were subsequently filled and his four colleagues, reassuring Jim all the time while holding him fairly firmly, Martin managed to gently break up the faeces and disimpact Jim's bowel. This was accompanied by Jim screaming invective at everyone. Martin says: 'After about half an hour, we rolled Jim onto his back, confident that we had performed an invaluable service. He sat up and spat at me.'

Enemas

'High, hot and a helluva lot!' was the phrase, or 'HHH' the acronym, written in the notes as instruction for an enema. Soap and water enemas were routine pre-operative preparation before bowel surgery in the 1960s and still going strong in the 1980s. David Barton, retired associate professor of nursing, says: 'The risk of perforating the bowel is horrifying to think of.'

Enemas were standard treatment for almost anything in the 1920s, as Margaret Broadley reports in *Patients Come First*. Four o'clock in the morning on a surgical ward was the set time for routine enemas and irrigation of colostomies. It's not clear when the optimal time was for sleep.

Castor oil was also given as a precursor to bowel surgery. In her nursing notes in 1924, Alice Clegg writes that to disguise the taste of castor oil, nurses should warm the glass in hot water, pour in a little lemon juice and brandy before adding in the castor oil, topping it off with a little more lemon juice.

Many of the rituals in nursing were driven by the demands of consultants and the bowel prep around Hartmann's procedure for a certain surgeon at Bart's in the 1980s was infamous. Hartmann's, where the latter part of the bowel is surgically removed, the anus closed off and a colostomy formed is used to treat colon cancer or severe inflammation of the bowel. Patients are usually in hospital for about 5–7 days, sometimes less if it is done as a laparascopic procedure. In the mid-80s patients were likely to be in for three or four weeks.

Admission, unlike today, was several days before the operation. At this time, the patient was allowed a light diet. This reduced to fluids and then clear fluids, such as water, black coffee, tea without milk, and finally on the night before the operation, no fluids. Bowel preparation involved giving a soap enema using the green soap delivered to the ward in a brown glass bottle. To further complicate the process, it was to be given as a rotating enema. This meant the patient had to roll from right side to left side, to front to back, all the while having three litres of warm soapy water poured through a funnel and orange tubing into their bowel. Not surprisingly, it wasn't unheard of for the contents of what you were pouring in to come gushing straight back out, often all over you if, like Judy, you weren't nimble enough to get out of the way: 'It was my birthday and I was meant to be going out that night!'

Patients had to hold onto the fluid for as long as possible but a commode was parked by the bed at the ready, armed with a stainless steel bedpan so that a maximum amount of noise reverberated around the ward from behind the curtains as they staggered from bed to commode.

Woe betide the poor nurse who, despite all her best efforts, there was faecal matter left inside the patient's bowel. Said surgeon would be straight on the phone yelling at the ward sister about the faecal contamination of his surgical field, demanding to know who the nurse was who failed to deliver a clean bowel.

Enemas were routinely given to women in labour until the 1970s. All kinds of reasons were given for this: it would reduce any soiling and the consequent embarrassment for women. It was also thought that by emptying the back passage there would be more room for the baby to be born and so reduce the length of labour and that it would cut any risk of infection to both the mother and the baby. It's not clear how much thought was given to the discomfort or indeed pain that an enema caused women. Increasingly, the voice of women in managing their own labour, together with studies demonstrating the lack of effectiveness of the practice, helped end this ritual.

To Kathy, it was all about the medicalisation of childbirth, turning pregnancy and labour into illnesses that had to be managed with medical intervention. She said it was a similar story in what were often called 'mothers' clinics' in the early 1970s, which were in fact contraception clinics – you had to be married to attend one and single women had to borrow a wedding ring to bypass this scrutiny. Women were called into see the doctor and to be weighed and have their blood pressure checked every three months, even if they had an intrauterine device (IUD) fitted. There was no evidence for the necessity of this, says Kathy, who points out that these days, contraceptive care is managed almost solely by nurses.

Severe wind can be very painful and often occurs after abdominal surgery. In 1924 Alice Clegg noted that Cajeput oil was given for flatulence, administered on a sugar lump. These days, peppermint water or tea is offered and once the patient starts to be up and about the wind soon dissipates. For those who are more incapacitated, a flatus tube can be passed into the lower part of the bowel and the other end is funnelled into a bowl of water releasing trapped wind and easing the patient's pain.

Rumour has it that at one time junior nurses were told to count the bubbles that emerged. It's not clear how many bubbles equalled success.

Turpentine, made from the distillation of resin from trees, has long been used for medicinal purposes because of its antiseptic properties. Available in Vick's VapoRub for example, and thankfully not as the product that we would recognise for cleaning or thinning paint. A turpentine enema encouraged a speedy and complete evacuation of the bowels. It was made by shaking up 1oz of turpentine with soft soap and water, followed by a pint of soapy water. Margaret remembers turpentine enemas being the post-operative normal in the 1920s for patients who were bloated with wind. She says: 'Two points were stressed, the turpentine must be mixed with several ounces of enema solution, and the patients anus and buttocks were well greased to prevent burning.'

An oil enema was given to soften hard faeces and done by injecting 3–5 oz of olive oil into the rectum, leaving for thirty minutes and then washing out with an 'ordinary' soap and water enema. A glycerine enema served much the same purpose and was a forerunner of today's simpler, glycerine suppositories.

Glucose saline enemas were given in an attempt to restore water and salts to the body when the patient couldn't eat or drink. These were administered slowly at body temperature.

Porridge enemas were the order of the day at St Mark's Hospital, London, one of the largest specialist bowel hospitals in the country. One nurse who worked there in the 1980s, remembers: 'We would give them to ladies with anal and rectal sphincter difficulties to test how strong their sphincter muscles were. When porridge or Ready Brek were not available then Weetabix was used instead.'

Constipation is quite often a feature of neurological conditions and milk and molasses, first gently warmed in a saucepan, was given via an enema to patients with raised intracranial pressure (pressure in the brain). The high sugar content of the molasses would soften hard impacted faeces and stimulate the bowel to work, while the osmotic effect of the sugar would help retain water in the colon, and so increase the natural action of the bowel.

With bodily fluids, there is always a risk of spilling bed pans or forgetting to turn off the valves on catheters allowing urine to quietly flood the floor. At Bart's we were taught to empty each catheter in turn into a jug which was discreetly covered with a paper towel as it was carried to the sluice, with always the fear that it might spill at any time. The less genteel but more efficient approach was to take a large bucket from bed to bed and empty the catheter at each stop. Obviously, this could only be done when measuring and testing of individual urines wasn't required. There was always a danger of slopping the urine as you staggered back to the sluice with a heavy bucket of the stuff.

While dealing with bodily fluids was part of the job, it didn't mean that you wouldn't rather avoid it. On a return to practice course – full of nurses remembering how it used to be and wanting to renew their registration – Karen remembers one saying that as a student she fumbled once with turning off a catheter valve and ended up with urine all over her hands. Seeing her aghast face, the senior nurse barked: 'Your hands are waterproof!'

Doris remembers nurses used to get quite down at having to manage the urinal washer:

> We used to forget which tap to turn and, if you turned on the wrong tap, a fountain would go to the ceiling and ruin your cap. That happened to dozens of us heaps of times. You were always turning on the wrong tap and you got drowned with the fountain from the urinal washer.

Over the years a range of different equipment for bedpans and urinals has been brought in. In the early days of course, these were made of china so woe betide the nurse who dropped one. As Margaret Broadley recounts, all breakages had to be paid for by the nurse herself. In *A Complete System of Nursing*, Millicent Ashdown recommends the 'Perfection' bedpan which had a larger opening than others and was easier to clean. As for urinals, she reports that glass was easier to clean than porcelain.

Much later, stainless steel bedpans came in and these could be put in giant washers, thus relieving nurses of the chore of washing them out and cleaning them. Dropping these made a terrible clang, drawing attention to the unfortunate nurse scuttling to the sluice with it, but at least it didn't break. Later still, papier mâché bedpans came into fashion and these could be placed in a plastic mould or in a commode and the whole thing then dispensed with in a bedpan masher. No cleaning required.

But modern isn't always good. Tom, later to become head of education at the RCN, remembers the early days at a new hospital in one of his first staff nurse roles.

> We soon realised that the bed pan mashers on the wards couldn't cope with the sheer volume that was being put through them and the drains were flooding out with faeces and papier mâché. We drove to a nearby hospital and snuck in and raided the wards for metal bedpans and stole away with them.

They went to one ward in particular because they knew the sister was something of a hoarder. A glance in a cupboard revealed boxes and boxes of war issue corn flakes. This was at least thirty-five years after the end of the Second World War. Eating those might well have sorted out anyone's bowel problems.

Chapter 7

Medicines and Mystical Powers

'Very few people had sleeping tablets, just a bedtime shot'

That heart-sink moment when you arrive home after a long shift only to find you have the ward keys in your pocket. And, in my case, trudging back two miles through rapidly deepening snow to return them to the ward.

For Kayte, it meant cycling back across London just as she had reached home, while others had a knock at the door from the local constabulary, prevailed upon to come and collect the keys – usually if someone had gone to bed and couldn't be woken by phone calls from the ward.

In keeping with hospital hierarchy, the key holder is the most senior nurse on the ward. Each staff nurse borrows the keys when she needs to administer drugs to her patients. Doctors do not get to hold the keys or have access to the controlled drugs cupboard.

There was one small bunch for the controlled drug cupboard and a larger bunch which featured all manner of keys including access to the regular drug cupboard, trolley and fridge. It was often weighed down with a block of wood which was meant to prevent people taking them home.

It always fascinated me why the regular bunch was so large. Often you would discover long redundant keys, for unused cupboards or doors to rooms long since converted into new bays. Mostly people had no idea what half of them were for. The advent of door key codes and swipe cards has slimmed this down in recent years.

You would think that it would be impossible to pop such a large bunch into your pocket and forget about them but believe me, you can. I arrived for a shift on a women's health ward when the weather was warm enough not to need a coat. By the end of the shift there was a foot of snow outside. I spent ages, clearing my car in the freezing cold, driving slowly home, skidding on the new snow, grateful to be getting home before the weather worsened, only to discover the ward keys in my pocket. Needless to say, the ward hadn't missed them but thought it hilarious that I had to trudge the two miles back as it wasn't safe to drive. You tell yourself you will never make that mistake again – but that was my second time!

As in the 'real world', the rules and our understanding around drugs in hospital are constantly changing. In the 1940s, nurses were informed that prescriptions should be written in Latin as this was the 'universal language'. They were also warned that doctors very often had poor handwriting (who knew?).

In the 1930s, Ann Lamb, a student at the Royal Infirmary Edinburgh, notes:

> The nurse is not responsible for either the drug or the dose ordered but is responsible for carrying out Doctors' orders. [You must] be able to report effect of [the] drug and know what sort of effect to look for.

These days nurses need to know the purpose of a drug and whether the dosage is appropriate. I'm not sure any nurse whatever the era would have gone ahead and given something they thought might be harmful.

Mary, who began her training in 1948, says that much of the learning they did was by rote so their actions were automatic. For medicine they learned the ditty:

> M is for medicine
> Read the label
> Shake it
> Take out the cork – no smell
> Measure it up
> And watch the patient take it

Drugs are only ever checked and given by a registered nurse. Over the decades drug rounds have been performed by first one then two nurses and now one again. It can be an art form making sure you are giving the right tablets to the right patient. The number of times a patient has obligingly agreed their name is Miss Smith when in fact it is nothing of the sort, always amazes me. There is certainly a lesson there in following procedure and always reading charts and name tags and then checking with the patient because all too often they are happy to oblige and be whoever you want them to be.

The drug assessment when we were training was one of four practical ward-based competencies that we had to pass. The others were total patient care, aseptic technique and ward management. For the drug assessment a clinical nurse tutor accompanied you on a drug round and assessed your competency and safety as you checked and measured out the drugs. I got in such a state with mine that the tutor asked me if I was left or right handed as I couldn't seem to decide which hand to hold a bottle and pour, and which one to hold the receptacle. Being naturally clumsy, I was terrified of dropping pills or spilling medicine.

Jacqui's drug assessment was more dramatic: 'I was feeling really unwell but sister gave me a real dressing down and told me to get on with it.'

Minutes into the drug round, Jacqui fainted and was taken to A&E where appendicitis was diagnosed and she was whisked off to theatre.

Many nurses are trained to prescribe medicines. In the UK, there has been something of a reluctance to recognise that with extended training all registered nurses could take on this responsibility, as they do in other countries. However, it is now being considered for the curriculum here. This will be something else that fundamentally changes the nature of nursing – from the days of Florence, when brow-mopping was pretty much all that was available – to the modern-day technicians that nurses are required to be.

In Mary's day, at the start of the NHS, drugs were checked by two nurses and you had to carry a big heavy tray full of bottles and pills around the ward in order to distribute them to patients. Then came magnificent trolleys with little compartments for each bed number. From the 1970s, drug trolleys could be taken around the ward (by one or two nurses depending on the rules at the time) and were locked and chained to the wall when not in use. Later, patients had their own bedside cabinet where their drugs were locked away. Now a computerised system means touchscreens and barcode scanning to identify patients and read their drug chart.

The modern process feels disconnected and no more efficient than previous methods. The patient's drug chart is no longer stored at the end of their bed. Instead, you log into a computer to see it. The computer is on a rather unwieldy set of wheels which can be taken to the patient's bed but this feels clumsy as you trundle back and forth between the treatment room where the ward drugs are stored, and the patient's bedside drug cabinet. Whoever designed the system didn't ask a nurse because no thought seems to have been given to the number of steps nurses need to take whenever a patient requires a drug.

Accessing controlled drugs – that is opioids such as diamorphine (heroin) for pain relief on a hospital ward has always been rather like one of those Russian dolls. Locked in a cupboard within a cupboard, within a locked room, checked and cross-checked before it can be administered. Historically, the requirement for two nurses to check controlled drugs has often meant a delay in patients receiving pain relief and that is still the case today. In a study by Mann and Redwood (2000), it was reported that patients generally waited about thirty minutes to get their pain relief.

Margaret Broadley remembers the dance required to give drugs on night duty in the 1920s:

> The staff nurse could give only the simplest drugs, such as aspirin, and the decision to give anything prescribed 'as required' rested with the night sister who was responsible for several wards at night so was never in one place. This meant that junior nurses spent much of the night chasing round the hospital looking for her, prescription board, bottle and spoon, or injection tray in hand. Once night sister had been located the medicine would be checked and the junior would make the perilous return journey often up or down five flights of stairs balancing the prescribed dose in the spoon. Watching the pills roll off the spoon into the dust or the liquid spill was always a possibility leading to a repeat of the exercise or a swift blowing off of the dust on the pills.

It was still a performance in the 1940s: Dorothy Carter (*Sisters*, Barbara Mortimer):

> I think it took at least ten minutes to give a quarter grain of morphia. We first had to get the glass syringe out of the spirit ... we had to rinse it out in cold water and then we took

the morphia from a minute vial, having counted it to make sure that the right amount of drug was there as recorded in the drug book. We took out one of the minute pills, like a· little saccharine pill, and put it into a teaspoon with water. That was then boiled up over a spirit lamp and drawn up into the syringe.

This then had to be carried to the patient, names checked, drug administered and then back to the treatment room to dismantle the syringe, wash it and sterilise it and sign the drug record book.

Opium and belladonna

Reference to opium and belladonna can be found in Greek mythology and they have been used for pain relief ever since. Opium is derived from the unripe seedpods of the opium poppy. Its use, by way of eating or drinking laudanum (opium in alcohol), was widely accepted in Victorian England. Dozens of formulae based on laudanum were sold as patent medicines for teething pain, colic, or even to keep children quiet. Opium use started to be regulated in the early twentieth century, first by pharmacists and then by doctors

In hospital, in the 1940s, opium could be applied on a soft cloth dipped in hot water, known as a stupe. A teaspoonful sprinkled on the stupe or flannel after it had been wrung out was applied to the skin. To counteract opium poisoning, 5–8oz of strong black coffee was given.

Sometimes a glycerine of belladonna was spread on a painful body part in a treatment known as a fomentation. In the notes of one nurse at Royal Infirmary Edinburgh in the 1920s, nurses had to be aware that some people were 'susceptible to the influence of belladonna', and they should note and report any dilation of the pupils or complaint of dryness of the throat, both symptoms that pointed to a 'slight degree of belladonna poisoning'. Belladonna is still used in medicines today in the treatment of Parkinson's disease, and for spasms of the gut such as irritable bowel, diverticulitis and infant colic. It is also useful for travel sickness as it reduces stomach secretions.

Mystical powers

Some potions were credited with an almost mystical power. The Brompton Cocktail was one of these. It was given for pain and as a 'pick you up' to patients who were terminally ill. Its ingredients varied slightly over the years and from hospital to hospital but essentially it consisted of morphine, alcohol and cocaine mixed with water and syrup and sometimes an anti-sickness drug. The Brompton Cocktail is thought to have derived from a mixture created by a surgeon, Herbert Snow, in the 1890s as a treatment for those who were terminally ill. Professor David Clark of the University of Glasgow, has a special interest in end of life care. According to his guide to the history of the Brompton Cocktail, such mixtures were established in the interwar years.

The idea was that the alcohol aided dissolution of the morphine and syrup made the concoction more palatable. We were certainly still administering it in the 1980s when I trained and I think we gave it with a sense of relief, knowing that the patient's pain would be controlled and that they would experience something of a 'feel good' factor.

Professor Clark says that the mixing of substances and liquids is a 'medicine of faith rather than fact', and perhaps that describes much of the ritual and myth in nursing – an instinct and faith for what works. Over time as we have become more knowledgeable, we have come to value evidence and apply it appropriately to care and treatment. It's clear that the careful balancing or titration of medicines today means a patient's pain can be more carefully and accurately controlled. The (very) gradual demise of the Brompton Cocktail can be seen as part of the move to evidence based medicine and a much greater sophistication in end of life care.

Bottoms up

It seems hard to believe in these days of alcohol awareness that not so long ago drug rounds also included beer, sherry and brandy, in little brown bottles, with bottles and cans of Mackeson's in the drugs cupboard as regular medicines. Alcohol for medicinal purposes was exempt from excise duties and had to be prescribed so that records could be kept. Jean recalls:

> In 1958 we took the drinks trolley round at 11:30 – to tempt the patients' appetites and up their iron levels. I got shouted at by an elderly patient on my first ward for not tipping the glass and pouring the Guinness slowly. They did not teach us that at PTS!

As recently as the 1970s, pregnant women were advised of the benefits of drinking Guinness and on the postnatal wards there was a pre-lunch Guinness trolley – to boost iron levels. On the vascular wards brandy and whisky were given to patients to encourage dilatation of the blood vessels and on plastics too but, observes one former nurse, 'generally, only to those who regularly drank.'

While another says: 'The patients used to love me doing the round, as I didn't have a clue about measures, I'd give them a tumbler full of whatever spirit they wanted!'

At St Bartholomew's Hospital, light ale was on the evening drinks trolley as a result of a Royal Charter which required the breweries in the City of London to provide for the hospital's patients; a practice still being adhered to until the late 1980s. Beer was given out most commonly on male surgical wards – perhaps to encourage men to drink more fluids. Sherry stimulates the appetite and was often prescribed for older patients before a meal. Sometimes brandy was prescribed and added to hot milk and sugar to aid sleep.

Mary Anne remembers that bedtime drinks on the drug trolley included sherry and whisky and there was also gin for any patient who couldn't pee post-operatively, if running the taps loudly didn't work. She says: 'Very few people had sleeping tablets, just a bedtime shot.'

Christmas was often liberally laced with alcoholic treats from the drugs trolley. One nurse remembers: 'Sister would go around with a fully laden trolley and dole out aperitifs. Then the consultant would carve.'

A roast turkey and all the trimmings were provided for patients and staff on the wards. This reflects a time when many patients were in hospital for longer periods and many over Christmas. Sue remembers one consultant – he of the bike leathers, 'used to always dress up as Santa at Christmas and go around the hospital on roller skates!'

Even those who couldn't eat and drink shared in the celebrations with pureed Christmas dinner and champagne brandy cocktails going down their nasogastric (NG) tubes.

Staff might also be the worse for wear. Many students, 18 years old and enjoying their first Christmas on the wards, were surprised to be greeted early in the morning with an offer of a drink from the trolley. One remembers her father coming to collect her after her shift finished at 15.00 on Christmas day and asking her if she was drunk as she clambered into the car. She was. Fortunately, staff numbers on the wards were high and while discipline was strict about a range of seemingly innocuous things, the mild intoxication of students during festivities was not regarded as serious.

Drinking was a part of life and so was smoking for much of the twentieth century. Kayte looked after one old lady – she of poo-rolling Malteser fame – who was brought in after causing a fire in her home because she was smoking under the bed covers.

It was almost mandatory for nurses to smoke, remembers Linda.

> The stench of cigarettes on us must have been disgusting for poor sick patients but I never remember any of them complaining, probably most of them smoked too. They used to sit in bed smoking, using the ashtrays on their lockers.

In the 1980s, although ashtrays were no longer a feature on patients' lockers, they still smoked in bed if they could get away with it. Usually, though, they collected on benches at the busy ward entrance, often only a few feet away from another patient relying on the life-saving supply from an oxygen cylinder!

Chest infections, exacerbated by smoking could be treated with antibiotics and once well again, people were able to forget how bad their cough had been, how painful their chest and were soon back on the fags, if they had ever stopped them.

The extent of heart disease and cancer caused by smoking was something we were well aware of in the 1980s, but somehow we failed to connect our all-important health role with helping people to stop. In those days there was very little around by way of smoking cessation services and people were just expected to quit. We didn't really understand the addictive nature of nicotine. Doctors and nurses continued to set a bad example with so many smokers among us. I remember going to see a GP soon after my mother died of lung cancer. He lit a cigarette in the consulting room. Needless to say, I didn't go back.

The arrival of antibiotics

The development of antibiotics revolutionised medical treatment, and the rituals of nursing care. Research into antibacterial medications began before the Second World War. One of the first sulphonamide drugs to appear was known as M&B 693, named after the manufacturers, May and Baker, which Mary remembers as a huge tablet that had to be taken morning and evening. One nurse, interviewed by Graham Thurgood for his thesis on a *History of Nursing in Halifax and Huddersfield 1870–1960*, remembers that until M&B 693 was available, there was virtually no treatment for the young men on her ward who were suffering from cerebrospinal meningitis. She describes how, intermittently three or four nurses had to gently hold down the young men so that cerebral spinal fluid could be released via a lumbar puncture. This practice rapidly became obsolete when the young men could be treated with the sulphonamide.

Another new drug was Prontosil, which Doris Carter remembers as being 'horrible stuff'. It was red and made the patient's skin red as well as colouring the glass syringes in which it was given. Other nurses from that era described penicillin, also administered by injection, as painful enough 'to make brave men cry'. In the 1940s penicillin was in powder form and might be stored in a pantry as there were no fridges. The powder was mixed with water prior to injection.

Penicillin was given in ways that today might be considered unconventional. At the Royal Infirmary Edinburgh (RIE) it was applied as a cream to burns and deep wounds and for wounds that were dry. A mixed sulphonamide-penicillin powder was blown directly onto the wounds using an insufflator and sometimes given dissolved in a mixture of beeswax and peanut oil or in a saline (salt) solution.

Working in theatres in the 1950s, Vera was finally allowed in close to see what was going on. She was given the penicillin powder spray and told to squirt it over the wound when it had been closed up. She squirted and a load of ants shot out. It's not clear who was blamed for this outrage but not surprisingly, Vera felt it was somehow her fault.

Infusion was considered one of the better methods of administering penicillin. At the RIE an apparatus – an early and rather complicated version of the drip infusions we see today – was used to run the infusion. It was the nurse's duty to refill the supply bottle each day, which was a move towards technology and away from the traditions of nursing care. Until then, fresh air and administering poultices to wounds and sponge baths to reduce high temperatures, were more or less the only treatment for infection.

Early on, penicillin use was greatly restricted, mostly due to its lack of availability and because the full extent of how effective it could be was unknown. Nurses in the early days decried the limited use of these wonder drugs – given as a last resort to the sickest patients while others with pneumonia and similar serious infections did without. It is said that Churchill was treated with the new wonder drugs in 1942 when severely ill with pneumonia. Penicillin was still only used in rare cases in the late 1940s.

Research has shown that the accuracy of the doses administered were also variable and it is likely that reduced strength doses of penicillin were being given. They may also have contained impurities which were a particular problem during wartime and which would have further weakened the dose. This 'under use' of an antibiotic can enable bacteria to build resistance to it more easily and it is quite possible that the antibiotic resistance that we talk of today may stem from the early days of penicillin use.

Since then of course there has been something of an antibiotics bonanza with these wonder drugs given out perhaps a little too frequently, enabling bacteria to build resistance to them. Aunt Molly's view, shared by many, is that an overreliance on clearing infections with antibiotics made people sloppy about good hygiene leading to some of the more modern-day problems of so-called 'hospital acquired infections'.

At one time in the 2000s, MRSA together with Clostridium difficile (C. diff) seemed to have taken hold of our hospital wards. Initially, most staphylococcus infections were sensitive to penicillin. But over time its repeated use led to many infections becoming resistant to penicillin and methicillin (a related drug developed to treat these bugs). Thus, the term methicillin-resistant staphylococcus aureus (MRSA) was derived.

Now a strict regime of testing patients for MRSA when they come into hospital, together with skin washes and antibiotic cream for the nasal passages (which can harbour MRSA) has started to get the infection under control. There is also a renewed awareness of good hygiene practice from hand-washing audits to check that professionals are washing their hands, to the deep cleaning of wards.

In the days when cleanliness was almost the only weapon nurses had against infection, handwashing in soap and water and various antiseptics was routine. For example, in Mary's time at the inception of the NHS, Mercury Perchloride Lotion was locked in the poisons' cupboard. It was tinted blue and regarded as a 'good disinfectant for hands when mixed to 1 in 1000 strength'. However, it was also described as 'one of the strongest poisons known'.

The introduction of new drugs often brings with it all kinds of restrictions and oversight. ACE inhibitors are an important group of drugs given to treat high blood pressure and to prevent strokes. They are usually prescribed by your GP who monitors their effect. When they were first introduced in the early 1980s, patients were often admitted overnight in order to supervise the first dose. In some ways it is reassuring that this level of care was taken.

As technology has advanced, nurses have moved into more technical care such as taking blood and inserting cannulae, so it is hard to believe that not so long ago, giving antibiotics was the job of the beleaguered house officer (F1 or F2 or first- or second-year doctor).

Equally, there are some procedures that we carried out without much thought for possible dangers that now require a specific training course before they can be undertaken. Inserting tubes into patients was a basic nursing skill in my student days. I remember learning to insert an NG tube (for the administration of liquid food and medicines for those who couldn't eat) quite early on in my training, finding I was efficient at it and so doing it many times over after that. When I returned to nursing in 2003, there were training and safety checks in place before anyone was allowed to insert an NG tube, as opposed to the slightly reckless hit and miss approach of my student days. More relaxed still is the 1940s version of *Modern Professional Nursing Vol II* which advises:

> Once the tube is in the stomach the patient will be less frightened (and it is not out of place to say that probably

81

the nurse will also be thankful) … Feed must be given asap but it is useless to start until all the inevitable coughing and spluttering is over.

Advice for stomach lavage (wash out) was also offered: 'Weak mustard and water may be used for alcoholics.'

Gail, who trained at St Thomas's Hospital in the late 1970s, remembers it being standard practice in A&E to perform gastric lavage on patients who had taken overdoses before a doctor had even seen them. This involved encouraging the patient to swallow a tube and administer liquid to clean out the stomach. 'I did that as a student nurse and never questioned the safety of what we were doing on any level,' she remembers now. 'I'm beginning to think that I was fortunate to get through my career without a disaster of some description!'

Chapter 8

Things that go Bump in the Night

'Since nature and authority dislike a vacuum, the time of the night
nurse was fully occupied making dressings, cleaning equipment,
testing urine, doing the flowers or any other tasks.'

When Susie learned during her interview for nurse training that she
would be required to work at night on the wards, she could only gasp:
'What all night?'

As it turned out, nights really didn't suit Susie. I remember she
and I were doing night shifts on opposite wards in our first year – hers
female surgical, mine male. When our respective colleagues went for
their breaks, we would sit with each other marvelling that the ward was
thought safe left in the hands of two 18-year-olds instead of one. Susie
was more anxious about this than I, who had not given much thought to
what might go wrong and what I would do if it did.

During our training we had to do twenty weeks of nights in the three
years – much less than previous generations but more than those who
came after. Eight weeks of night duty in three years was the norm by the
mid-1980s.

For Linda at the Manchester Royal Infirmary (MRI) in the 1960s, the
night shift lasted twelve hours and was worked in three-month blocks.
Each ward had thirty-two patients and was staffed by two nurses – a
'senior', who was only a second- or third-year student nurse and a junior
or runner, who was a first-year student nurse. The junior nurse was left
on her own for half an hour, while her more senior colleague went for a
break. Linda says:

> For a first-year nurse, it was a terrifying experience to be
> left alone with 32 sick patients. There were also the ghosts
> to contend with. The ghostly sister who came and tapped

83

you on the right shoulder if you began to fall asleep and the nurse whose lower body could not be seen because she was walking at the level of where the original old floor had been.

One night, Linda's senior colleague had gone for her break when she heard a commotion in the side ward. On investigation, she found a confused elderly gentleman attempting to climb over the cot sides to get out of bed. Linda says:

> I tried to calm him. and offered to make him a cup of tea. He told me that he was going home. A very inexperienced 18-year-old, I told him that he was in hospital, it was the middle of the night and he couldn't do this. He became more agitated and stood up in the bed trying to put his leg over the cot side. Fearful that he would fall I tried to push his leg back and he, no doubt thinking that I was attacking him, put his hands around my throat in a vice like grip. He was amazingly strong. I was 5' 2" and weighed 7½ stone. I tried to prise his hands from my neck, he called me some choice names then let me go, climbed over the end of his bed and exited the room.

Linda ran to block his way as he headed towards the ward door but he spied the fire hose, uncoiled it and fired it at her, full blast. At that moment, the senior nurse appeared. He turned the hose on her and continued to drench them both from head to toe. Somehow, they managed to wrestle the hose from him and then, shivering and dripping, tried to cajole him into returning to his bed. Linda says: 'He was striking out at us and one of us managed to get to the phone to summon sister. She arrived, took in the situation and called the doctor.'

Eventually the patient was persuaded to return to bed and the doctor gave him an injection of paraldehyde, and within minutes he was calm and sleeping. Paraldehyde had a pungent aroma which hung in the air for hours after administration. The senior nurse and Linda were then told to go to the nurses' home and change into dry uniforms while sister looked after the ward.

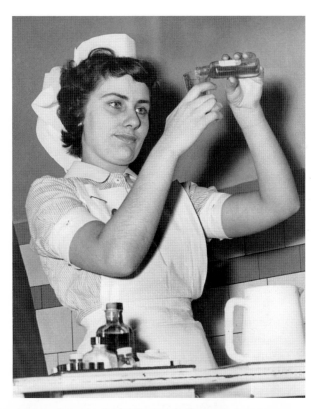

Nurse from Glasgow Royal Infirmary 1967. (The Herald and Times Group)

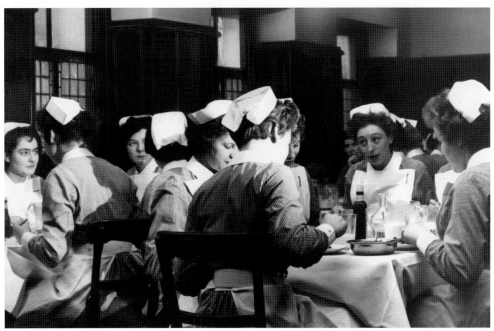

Nurses' dining room Western Infirmary Glasgow 1960s. (Copyright NHS Greater Glasgow and Clyde Archives)

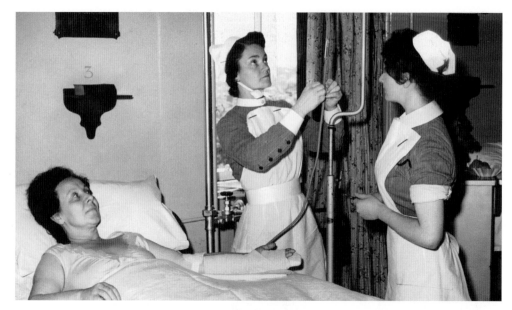

Setting up a blood transfusion; Western Infirmary, Glasgow 1960s. (Copyright NHS Greater Glasgow and Clyde Archives)

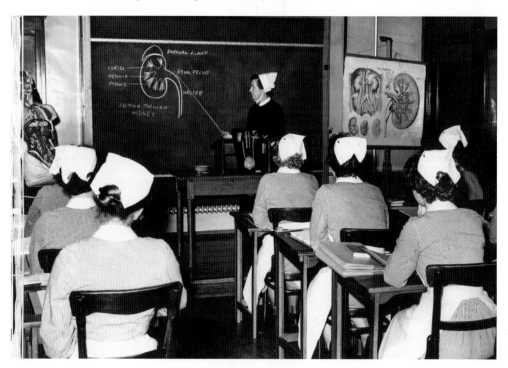

Student nurses in lecture 1960s Western Infirmary, Glasgow. (Copyright NHS Greater Glasgow and Clyde Archives)

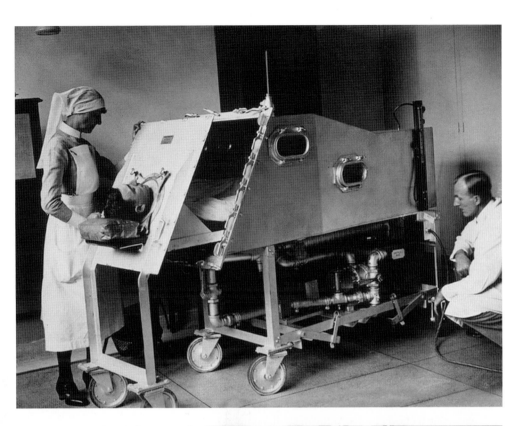

Above: Patient being nursed in an iron lung. (Wellcome collection)

Right: Student nurse St Helier Hospital, Carshalton, 1943. (Wellcome collection)

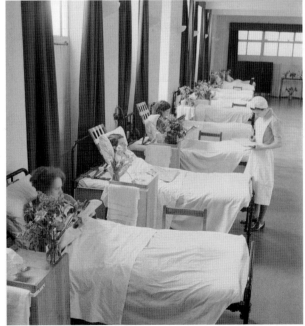

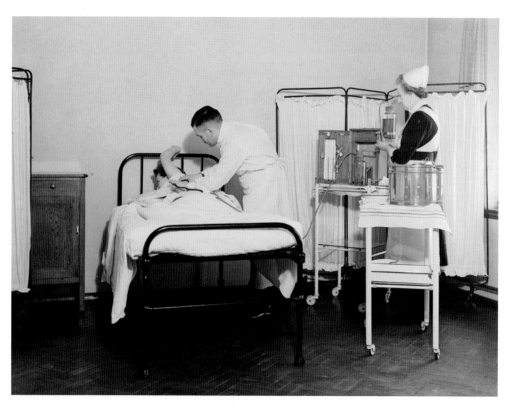

Inserting a chest drain. (Wellcome collection)

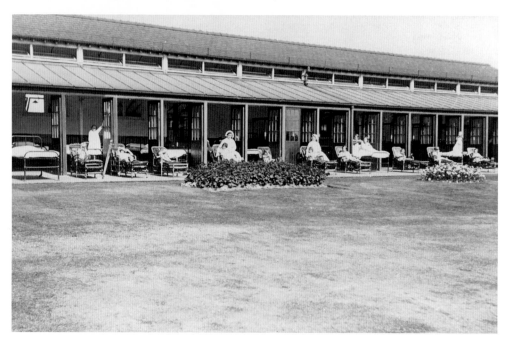

West Midlands Sanatoria. (Wellcome collection)

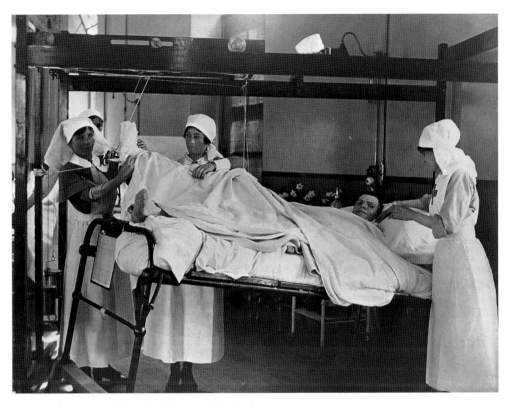

Patient in traction. (Wellcome collection)

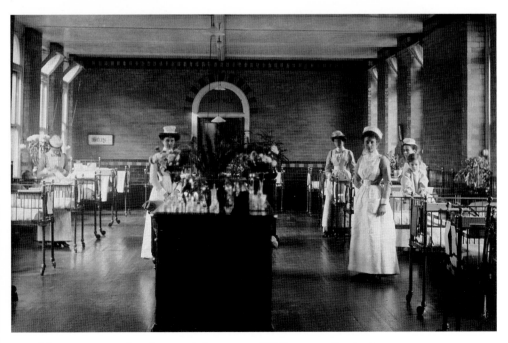

Nurses on a ward early twentieth century. (Wellcome collection)

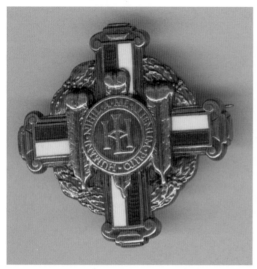

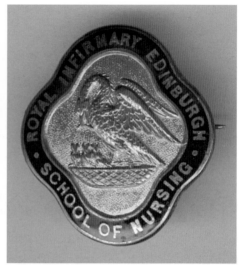

Above left: London Hospital badge. (RCN Archives 2015)

Above right: Royal Infirmary Edinburgh School of Nursing. (RCN Archives 2015)

Below left: Manchester Royal Infirmary badge 1973. (RCN Archives 2015)

Below right: Glasgow Royal Infirmary badge.

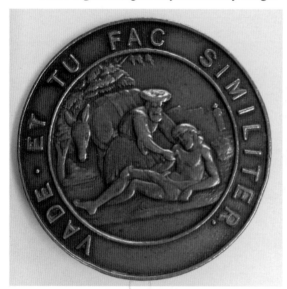

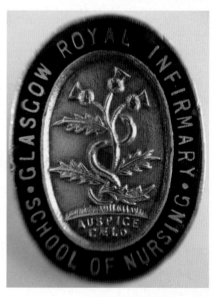

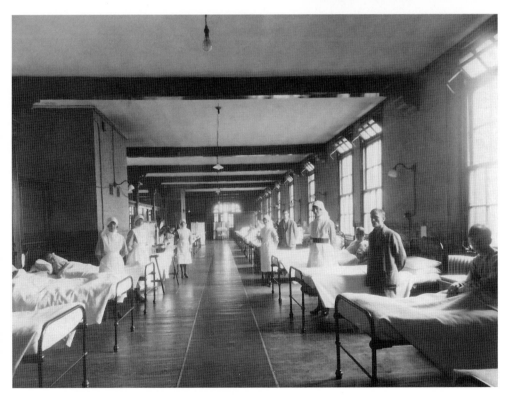

Right: Sam Gamgee who in 1880 invented Gamgee tissue, an absorbent cotton wool and gauze surgical dressing.

Below: E3 ward Hope Hospital, Salford 1927. Alice Clegg first on left. (Courtesy of Rosalind Gooley)

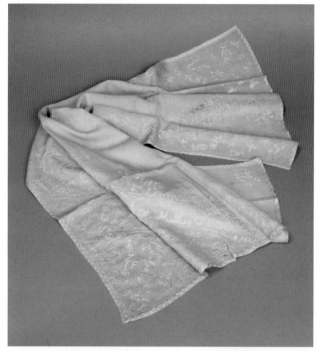

Headscarf embroidered with the initials of nurses who wore it when they were operated on by surgeon Mr James Sherren at the London Hospital. (Copyright Barts Health NHS Trust Archives and Museum)

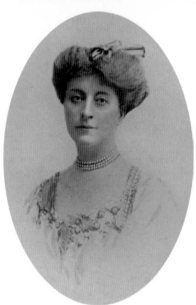

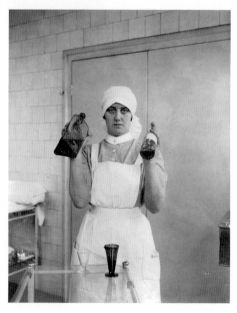

Above left: Nurse No. 1 Ethel Gordon Fenwick. (Courtesy Barts Health NHS Trust Archives and Museum)

Above right: All kinds of medicines and mixtures made it onto the drug trolley circa 1920s. (Copyright Barts Health NHS Trust Archives and Museum)

We were to do so as quickly as possible and then come back and mop up the water. I didn't get any lunch that night! The elderly gentleman recovered and was a delightful old man. He had no recall of the events.

Night sister seems to have been a fairly scary persona wherever you worked. Linda remembers her visiting the ward three times during the night. About 22.00, 02.00 and 06.00, depending on the needs of other wards. The senior ward nurse accompanied her on these rounds, stating name and diagnosis of each patient. You had to know all patients' names and diagnoses by the first visit at 22.00 even if you had arrived on the ward for the first time two hours earlier.

Very often night sister would have a penchant for knowing a particular fact about the patients. Often this would be their religion – perhaps because death often occurred at night and it was important that the correct religious and cultural rituals were followed. One night sister always wanted to know religion and who was on a potassium infusion. The latter presumably because of the health risks posed by potassium fluids going through too rapidly in the days before electric pumps monitored their throughput. The former, presumably in case this happened.

The wards were often cold but cardigans and hot drinks made the long nights bearable. Of course, both were banned – under the claim that it looked 'unprofessional' (although who could see in the dark) – so cardigans were hastily removed and cups, carefully balanced inside the top drawer of the desk, should night sister appear, silent as a cat. There was of course the night sister who was all too familiar with that routine and would purposefully slam the drawer shut. Not easy explaining the spilt contents and ruined paperwork to the ward sister in the morning.

Those wilier than me would scatter a little sugar or cereal near the ward doors so the crunch underfoot could be heard and give warning of night sister's approach. For those who worked at Hill End Hospital in St Albans, night sister's arrival was heralded by her cycling down the long corridors of what was once a huge mental health asylum. There's no record of whether she sounded a bicycle bell but anything was possible. Other nurses recall whizzing up and down the corridors on roller skates.

While night sister's visits tended to be a double-edged sword, some achieved legendary status: One New Year, Jacqui and her colleagues, popped a teddy bear in an empty bed complete with an intravenous infusion taped to his arm, ready to hand over to the day staff. Unexpectedly, night sister paid an extra visit to the ward. Jacqui says: 'She stopped in front of the bed with the teddy bear in and looked at me and said "this patient has not been turned since my last round".'

Socialising while on a nightshift was a no-no, so Gill was highly anxious when night sister asked to be taken round the ward just as Gill's colleague was taking her break with two friends, chatting in the day room. Cautiously, Gill accompanied night sister on her tour, unsure whether to take ages with each patient, giving her colleagues time to escape or to speed things up to get sister off the ward quickly. As you would expect, night sister went at her own brisk but thorough pace, even checking the quality of Gill's cleaning in the bathroom, glancing at the big red mackintoshes used during bed baths which were drying over the side of the bath, before exiting the ward. At which point there was a commotion from the bathroom as the red mackintoshes were thrown aside and the three nurses climbed out!

Leaving the hospital at night during a shift, albeit during your break, must also have been a no-no, so what possessed me to offer to go and collect a Chinese takeaway for myself and colleagues while working a night shift on the hospital's notorious Harvey ward – location of both a ghost and the robust Sister Harvey? Fortunately, I didn't bump into either as I took several backstreet alleys and shortcuts to a newly opened Chinese takeaway. As my colleagues and I tucked in we were all slightly gobsmacked at my audacity.

Remembering a generation earlier at the Manchester Royal Infirmary, Linda says:

> I have come to realise that we were treated very well at MRI in comparison to some other hospitals. When we wakened in the evening, we went to the special night nurses dining room and had breakfast. The dining room remained open and we had a cooked meal in the middle of the night and a cooked dinner when we went off duty at 08.00.

Imposter

The real godsend on nights, at least at Bart's, were registered nurses known as flashbelts. So called because they carried a bleep on their belts that flashed red when it went off. They were allocated an area of the hospital to cover for the night, supporting the night staff who were almost all students and responding to urgent need if they were bleeped. Their presence was comforting and I was in awe of their confidence and competence. They were usually young and friendly and not stiff and scary like night sister.

Alison worked as a flashbelt in the early 1980s for six months. One night, she was covering the surgical block and her first port of call was the busy female surgical ward on the ground floor. There were many sick and dependent patients who had undergone extensive colorectal surgery. Alison was there to administer controlled drugs for analgesia or palliation and antibiotics. She spoke to the third-year student who was in charge, well supported by her junior.

The house officer, Chris, was handing over to a locum. Alison returned at 22.00, the ward lights were down and the students, although busy, were in control. The house officer, Chris, was still handing over to the locum. He would have been on duty nearly forty-eight hours by then so it was odd to see him taking his time with handover. An hour or so later, Alison was summoned to the night office. Walking fast, never running, she arrived at the door in the basement, caught her breath, knocked and went in. The atmosphere was tense.

It seemed that the locum was an imposter. Not a doctor at all. Chris had twigged this and was staying close to him while alerting his colleagues. Not so easy in the days before a quick text even existed. Alison was deployed back to the surgical wards on the ground floor and kept an eye out for the imposter while doing that ubiquitous nursing ritual of tidying the linen cupboard. Doors from there opened into the ward and into the main corridor so she had a good view.

All the porters were manning the entrances and exits to prevent an escape. Six officers from the City of London Police, plus a police van were stationed outside A&E. Quietly, while being shown the 'on call' room, the imposter was arrested. Chris, the house officer and hero of the hour, eventually got home and his registrar was summoned to come in and cover. What became of the imposter is not known and in the days of no social media the story remained under the radar.

Endless tasks

Exciting encounters with imposters and scary levels of critical patients aside, night duty was also the home of endless tasks. These were the jobs that bookended the start and finish of nights. Monica Baly writing in *Nursing and Social Change* says this is down to when surgical patients were traditionally likely to stay three weeks or more and medical patients were bed bound for up to six weeks with infections or similar at a time when there were no antibiotics. As Monica says, 'Since nature and authority dislike a vacuum, the time of the night nurse was fully occupied making dressings, cleaning equipment, testing urine, doing the flowers or any other tasks.'

At the beginning of the night, many wards insisted that all flowers were removed and placed in the day room on the pretext that flowers sucked oxygen out of the air and this was dangerous at night. I have no idea where this myth came from but the result was you were less likely to knock them off the locker in the dark while administering to a patient. At the other end of a night shift there was such a long list of jobs to be done before morning, including returning flowers to their rightful owner, that very often these got underway not long after the evening staff left the ward.

While there is no succession of doctors' rounds or patients' visitors, wards are still pretty noisy places at night. It's hard to know how patients recuperate with so little sleep, sharing a room with more than thirty other people, subjected to a routine they have never experienced before.

Anything that needs checking is checked on nights – this includes controlled drugs, the resuscitation trolley and the blood glucose meter. These are vital routines to ensure equipment is working whenever it is needed. The rationale for why other checks were done at night was less clear. On one cardiothoracic ICU, patients had to be weighed between 03.00 and 05.00. With sixteen patients and one old sling scale, it was tough to get all the weights done because by 06.00 specimens were being collected for testing in the lab as well as the million and one other things that needed to be done to ensure the ward was shipshape for the morning staff. No one knew why the weights had to be done at that time other than it had always been that way.

Eventually someone discovered that the scale was shared with another ward who traditionally always had it from midnight to 03.00 before it moved to the next ward who had it from 03.00 to 06.00. No scientific reason just simple logistics.

One of the most important night-time jobs was collecting in the water jugs. I never did understand why this had to be done at night because it was impossible to do quietly. Fluid charts had to be added up to see how much patients had taken in and urinated out over the twenty-four hours. Although there were columns on the chart to complete, there didn't seem to be a failsafe method of recording intake and output.

Some nurses recorded a 1 litre bag of fluid as they set it up, some once it had finished. Cups of tea and glasses of water were 150mls except when they were 200mls or even 250mls. Added to which, patients invariably drank a bottle of Lucozade that they forgot to tell you about. Some wards were more organised and gave patients a graduated jug and if they had a cup of tea, the empty cup was supposed to be filled with water from the jug, so how much they had drunk could be deduced from reading the markings on the jug. Invariably someone would forget this rigmarole so the accuracy of the fluid balance charts was always in doubt.

The ward sister who insisted that fluid charts be completed in Roman numerals summed up the very essence of nonsensical ritual. No one could add up the numbers and most people only had a sketchy knowledge of how to write them.

Just as the regular observations of temperature, pulse and blood pressure often continued to be checked even when the patient's condition didn't demand it, so a fluid chart continued to be maintained for a patient for no apparent reason other than it was something that could be measured. For Michael, this was where the nursing process came into its own.

The nursing process was first described in the late 1950s but was still being introduced when I trained in the 1980s. The process took a scientific approach to nursing, working through five separate steps: assessment, diagnosis, planning, implementation and evaluation, to ensure patients specific needs were catered for and to improve the overall quality of patient care. The focus was on assessing each patient individually and planning and delivering their care accordingly, rather than subjecting everyone to the same routine. It was the start of the end of many of nursing's rituals.

Nights were often an opportunity to chat with a patient over a cup of tea and hear their worries and fears. I remember making tea for men who couldn't sleep and listening to their fears, now that they had survived a heart attack. At that moment they were ripe for information about keeping fit and well, and I regret that I knew so little – prevention of cardiovascular disease through diet and exercise featured so little in our education at that time. Those conversations stayed with me and influenced my later decision to study public health.

After the bewitching hour of 03.00 – which science has shown is when humans are at their lowest ebb and certainly one of the commonest times for deaths in a ward – morning approached all too rapidly and there was so much to do. Margaret Broadley recounts in *Patients Come First* that routine washing of patients in the 1920s began at 04.00, but also at this time there were four-hourly dressings to be completed, colostomy irrigations to be done and, of course, enemas to be given.

At the RIE in the 1960s, nurses were not allowed to wake patients before 06.00, but all thirty-two had to be washed by the time the day shift started at 07.30. On a medical ward with most patients on bedrest this meant the night staff had to stealthily start washing patients or handing out basins at about 05.00 so as to have everything done in time. Keen to get the work done, one junior nurse washed a patient's face and hands before realising she was dead.

At one time, a nurse working nights on a surgical ward would have to prepare theatre and attend the operation if a patient was admitted to the ward needing surgery. Evelyn Davies, whose story is recorded in the RCN's oral history collection, trained in Bridgend 1947–51. On night duty, if someone came in for surgery, she would leave the ward and lay up in theatre. This meant oiling up all the instruments, turning out a laparotomy set as standard for almost all operations and laying up the trolleys. She would stay to see the patient having the operation and wheel him back to the ward with the porter to help. Evelyn would then have to go back to theatre to boil the instruments ready for the next day. She also had to clean the theatre, which was hard work and, with the theatre being some distance from the general wards, more than a little scary at night.

Ghostly encounters

Hospitals are big places and the old ones have a mass of underground corridors and old fashioned lifts, provoking a plethora of ghostly stories and encounters with imposters of a different kind. Every hospital has a ghost, sometimes several, but usually it is a young woman who died in tragic circumstances.

Perhaps there is a need to believe in ghosts and an afterlife when hospitals are so closely associated with death. Nurses in particular have to cope with life and death on a daily basis and most of us fear making a mistake or feeling overwhelming if guilty relief when an error turns out to be someone else's fault. Very much a case of 'there by the grace…' etc. As already described, it was routine to leave two students in charge on a ward of up to thirty patients at night. We were so young and inexperienced, we often wondered how we survived, never mind the patients. However, ghosts can be great levellers.

Liz remembers night sister being particularly stern as she assessed her knowledge of a patient, when an unprogrammed cardiac monitor bleeped into action in the next bed. Wordlessly, the night sister turned on her heel and, Liz says, 'we didn't see her again that night'.

Most hospital ghosts are women – usually former nurses who offer help or warn of danger. They are often described as 'the grey lady', which might reflect the uniform of many years ago. Sister Thistlewaite was the resident ghost at St Mary's Hospital, London. Her portrait hung high on a wall in the hospital. Cate, says:

> She'd take bedpans from patients and we'd hear the bedpan washer go on but not see her. If a drip had gone through, the next bag of fluid would fall on the floor. If drugs were due, the drug chart would appear open at the end of the bed.

Kayte remembers two ghosts, one good, one bad, from her nursing days: 'I loved the ghost on ward six south at Charing Cross who used to come and keep you company in the common room during breaks on night duty.'

Very often though, ghosts portend death. On the first floor of the old University College Hospital (UCH) cruciform building, there was a wooden cabinet with shutters, behind which was the portrait of long-deceased surgeon Marcus Beck. As part of a nightly ritual, the night sister had to close the shutters and it was the day sister's duty to open them in the morning. If the shutters were not closed at night, then it would mean someone would die unexpectedly. Given the chances of an unexpected death in a large hospital at night, it's not clear just how much weight this ritual carried.

The ghost of nurse Lizzie Church is also said to haunt UCH. Reputedly Lizzie had mistakenly given a patient – who apparently was also her fiancé – an overdose of morphine when she was still training and was so traumatised by her error that she killed herself. Thereafter her ghost hovered over any nurse administering morphine to a patient.

The philosopher Jeremy Bentham was preserved in the form of an 'auto icon' at University College London after his death and the dissection of his body by his friend, the surgeon Thomas Southwood Smith. The auto icon consists of his skeleton covered by a 'body' made of straw and other materials, dressed in his finest clothes and topped by a wax likeness of his head. It's on display in a glass case at University College London. His ghost has apparently been seen wandering the corridors, while others have heard the tapping of his walking-stick (which is on display in the glass case with him).

As a student at St Thomas's Hospital, London, Mary Anne received direct help from the hospital's ghost. Nursing a distressed elderly woman who was dying, Mary Anne left her to fetch some water from the kitchen opposite, only to return to a calm and smiling woman sitting up in bed on freshly plumped pillows. The patient said she had been helped by the lady in the grey dress. Mary Anne hadn't spotted anyone going into the room in the moments that she was away and her colleagues said that none of them had been into help the patient.

The patient died later that evening still calm and smiling. This was Mary Anne's first experience of death and the ward sister asked how she was coping. Mary Anne says:

> I explained what had happened, including the strange reference to a lady in grey and said that as the patient had calmed down and seemed at peace that made me feel much happier about it. Sister sat back in her chair and told me the story of the Grey Lady.

A young student nurse (possibly a nun) had been left to look after a patient who was agitated. The nurse left the patient alone and the patient had an accident and died. The young nurse was distraught and threw herself off the stairwell to her death and her ghost appears to patients who are agitated, especially before they die. The old-fashioned uniform at the hospital was a long grey dress.

Similar stories of young nurses killing themselves as a result of a perceived failing include the Pink (junior sister) at Bart's who mistakenly caused a patient's death when she gave them the wrong drug. She later made her ghostly presence felt by tapping nurses on the shoulder when they were administering drugs and reportedly about to make a mistake. Alternative versions of this are that she whispers in the nurse's ear, 'check again, check again'. Similarly, Linda remembers a ghost from her days at Manchester Royal Infirmary: 'A ghostly night sister patrolled the wards ready to tap the shoulder of any nurse who dozed off.'

At the former Mothers' Hospital, in Hackney, East London, drowsy nurses also complained of feeling a tap on the shoulder. According to legend, a nurse who was bottle-feeding a newborn baby dozed off and slumped forward in her sleep, smothering the baby. Full of remorse, she killed herself and was condemned to walk the wards, tapping young nurses on the shoulder to keep them awake.

I spent three months at the Mothers' Hospital for my obstetrics placement. It was a strange place run by the Salvation Army which left me with quite an antipathy towards the Sally Army. Among other things, I disliked the adherence to daily prayers which they imposed on the women, most of whom were very poor and disadvantaged and needed more than prayers. The youngest mother I met was 13 years old, accompanied by her mother and siblings. As a student, without knowledge of what might be going on in terms of child protection (probably very little in the 1980s), it seemed to me that prayers might be said but eyebrows were barely raised.

I felt immensely privileged to witness childbirth – to realise that suddenly there was another human being in the room but I was completely spooked by the freezer room for placentas. It was invariably the student nurse's job to take the placenta, once it had been checked by the midwife, to the freezer.

The door to the room of the freezer operated on auto-close and I hated it if the door closed behind me so I used to balance on one leg trying to keep the door open while opening the freezer and depositing the placenta, panic rising when I couldn't manage these acrobatics. I'm not sure what I thought would happen but I knew I didn't want to be in that room any longer than necessary.

And then there was murder: At St Bartholomew's Hospital there was supposedly a ghost of a lady who cried by the fountain in the hospital square after throwing her baby out the window, while the lift in the hospital's Queen Elizabeth II block (now demolished) was legendary. Sometimes known as the 'coffin lift', nobody but nobody would use it at night. Set within the stairwell, when you pressed the button, if it came at all, it would take you to the basement and the lights would go out. If you chose the stairs, the lift doors would open at every floor as you reached it – although there would be no one inside.

So many people reported this experience that it was simply accepted. The story was that a nurse had been murdered by a patient from the neurology ward in the lift and she continued to haunt it. In another part of the hospital, also in a lift, a doctor claimed to have seen the ghost of a nurse in uniform including a hat – at a time when hats were no longer part of the uniform. Was he hallucinating after a punishing shift or was this another ghost haunting another lift?

We often think of ghosts floating along and some have put this down to the changes in floor levels in a building over centuries. For example, the ghost of Rahere, the twelfth-century founder of Bart's is said to haunt the hospital and floats above floor level. And at Glasgow Royal Infirmary, a ward sister was thought to have floated along, visible only from the knees up; it was the same for the ghost at the MRI.

The Royal College of Nursing (RCN) building on Cavendish Square in London has its own ghost. In 1883, Jane Elizabeth Barrington, Viscountess Barrington of Ardglass, was killed by an 'accidental' fall on the beautiful painted staircase at 20 Cavendish Square. You can still see the black square on the fifth step from where she fell. Her husband reportedly placed a silver cross on this stair in her memory which has since been removed, with only some repair work left to show. Her ghost – the 'grey lady' – has supposedly been seen stalking the corridors ever since.

Chapter 9

Dust, Dirt and Domesticity

'Dust is dirt and dirt is disease, possess yourself of a duster,
and follow me.'

Cleaning, and above all cleaning *properly,* was pretty much the core of being a nurse for most of the first half of the twentieth century. Cleanliness and the role it played in reducing the risk of the spread of infection dates back to Florence Nightingale, although paradoxically Florence did not believe that nurses should be cleaning. In the Harley Street Institution for the Care of Sick Gentlewomen in Distressed Circumstances established by her, she introduced quite revolutionary labour-saving devices – lifts and piped hot water so nurses could nurse and not clean. She wrote: 'to scour was a waste of power'.

Unfortunately, those who set up the early nurse training schools had different views and that, together with the overdeveloped sense of discipline, remained the nurse's lot for many generations. Somehow keeping a ward tidy and clean was connected to the very morality of the nurse.

One nurse reported from the Royal Infirmary Edinburgh (RIE):

> Dusting is the first thing to be done in a ward. This may seem to many to have v little to do with nursing but we must remember that the air is filled with small particles of dust and although invisible they are always present.

In pre-NHS days beds were often donated to the hospital by local benefactors and a brass plate would go up on the wall above the bed celebrating the donation. Margaret says: 'Your first job in the morning wasn't the patient, it was cleaning the brass plates.'

With a probationer each side of the long ward, you could race against each other to see who would finish the brass plates on their side first.

In the early days there was a tendency to think of nurses simply as nicely brought up, well-educated servants. Their uniform was designed around that worn by servants and many women from the servant classes also did private nursing. The profession has grown from these origins, but the importance of good hygiene to protect the patient (and the nurse) and promote good health is still necessary, if less easily managed. It is good that nurses are no longer expected to do basic cleaning, but a clean ward is still an essential part of good care.

Cleaning in theatres took up a huge part of nurses' time. Alison remembers:

> Students and qualified nurses did all the cleaning – except for the floor. Staff nurses did a spirit round of all horizontal surfaces and students washed the walls – all of them – with a Spontex mop and Teepol on a late shift at the end of the day. It was totally exhausting to do this properly but I understand infection rates were low!

These days, cleaners are almost always outsourced from a private company and no longer employed directly by the NHS. They may have little connection to the ward or theatre, a link that can be vital in a pressured environment when action is needed quickly.

In an interview for the RCN oral histories, Alice Kemp, who began her training in 1918 just as she turned 21 years old, remembers how unkind some of the ward sisters were and says:

> I had my own back on one sister. They had a water room where they threw all the dirty linen and you had to sort it out. They had a stand pipe with a big brass handle and a big brass thing on top that you had to clean. I was cleaning this one day and, in the reflection, I saw the sister standing watching me in the doorway waiting for the doctors' rounds so I thought well I'm having my own back time. I will just push this lever and it shot clean out straight into her best white cap!

Margaret Lamb trained in the 1930s: 'We had to have all the incontinent patients' clothes washed before they went to the laundry. They had to be sluiced first then they went into a bag and were taken away.'

Soiled linen was not dried on the ward as it caused an unpleasant smell. All infected clothes were wrung through carbolic acid before being sent to wash.

Basic laundry and domestic cleaning formed a large part of Mary's day in the 1940s. She also remembers being pushed headlong into a bath full of dirty laundry by a passing patient, which she regarded as just one of the hazards of being a nurse:

> We spent a lot of time cleaning blood and faeces off sheets. Everything was wet washed before it went to the laundry. The night staff would soak the sheets in the bath and we would rinse them out and put them in bins ready for collection. It sorted us out – whether we could cope with it or not. I guess that's why they did it.

Evelyn reports: 'It was known as "slunging" in Edinburgh in the sluice room. We got some extremely disagreeable, nasty, dirty jobs to do,'

The first job of the day for the most junior student nurses at MRI was to fill the foul linen bin – large dustbins which were filled with water and disinfectant. Soiled and contaminated linen went in there. Filling with water by hose was extremely slow and so the hapless nurse would leave it to fill while she got on with other duties. Inevitably the bin would overflow, causing much consternation and more work.

Michael did a combined training of general and mental health nursing in the 1960s. As a student he was locked in with the psychiatric patients on the ward, while the charge nurse and staff nurse were doing administrative tasks in the office. 'These patients had various levels of distress but I worked out that distressed patients were really quite good at working with me at cleaning the toilets!'

Twelve chapters in *Modern Professional Nursing New and Revised Edition Vol II* are devoted to hygiene. One concentrates solely on ward cleanliness with clear descriptions of how a ward should be cleaned – all the beds pulled out from the wall and the dust swept towards the door, keeping the broom low so as to prevent the dust from flying about. It was the nurses who pulled out the beds to clean behind them and it was the nurses who used their own scissors, bought with their own money, to scrape the dirt off the wheels of the beds.

Angela remembers in the 1950s that high and low dusting was done before breakfasts were given out and then tea leaves were scattered on the floor to collect up the dirt before sweeping. A ritual that had been in place for the best part of the previous fifty years.

According to 1940s *Modern Professional Nursing*: 'the ward floor is usually the pride of the entire staff.... Wooden parquet floors are polished with special mops or electric polisher ... this is to prevent the growth of organisms which do not thrive on a dry shiny surface.'

There is even advice on flowers: flower vases need to be washed daily and filled with clean water and the flowers freshly arranged each morning. Nowadays, of course, flowers are generally banned from hospital wards on the grounds of infection risk although it's not quite clear what risk they pose, except perhaps if someone has an allergic reaction to them.

However, it is much easier to provide care without risk of knocking them off the locker as you push back the curtains, or of the flowers staining your clothes – lilies being the worst culprits (Sellotape placed over the top of the stain and ripped off usually gets the stain out).

Locker rounds were a daily routine. Going round with the ubiquitous trolley and a bowl of warm water, nurses cleaned all the lockers and washed the ashtrays – standard issue at one time – chatting with patients, something that was not encouraged unless you were also completing a task. As the daughter of a nurse this was all very familiar. The efficiency and method of cleaning was transferred to the home and I learned all about damp dusting long before I became a nurse myself. It was many years before I realised that not everyone approached their housework with quite the same vim and discipline!

Recently, some hospitals have brought in the concept of 'intentional rounding,' whereby a nurse goes round the ward every hour to ask each patient how they are and to check if they need to use the toilet or to have a drink. Many in the profession scoff at this new ritual, saying such checks were an automatic part of nursing care and should not have needed to be formalised.

Intentional rounding is less about chatting with patients and more about ensuring the absolute basics of care have been offered. For Martin, training as a psychiatric nurse, chatting with patients was at the core of his work and so when called upon to apply his particular skills while doing his general nursing placement, he couldn't refuse.

He was despatched to the surgical ward to help with a patient who was experiencing post-anaesthetic confusion. As Martin recalls:

> A rather large policeman who had no idea if it was Thursday or Regent Street, kept trying to get out of bed and was seriously intent on thumping anyone who came near. I was sent into his side room with the words: 'You're psychy, you'll know what to do.' I didn't have a clue.

Martin says:

> It is a commonly held belief that psychiatric hospitals and units are overflowing with aggressive, hostile and dangerous people who would rather kill you than smile but my experience, gained through 12 years of practice, is almost the opposite... I rarely encountered any kind of hostility and had never been hit in the line of duty so a beefy copper with a grievance against the world was completely outwith my experience or training.

As Martin went into the patient's room, he raised his hands in surrender to show he meant no harm and the burly policeman seeing he wasn't being opposed, sank back on his pillows. That, or the fact that at over 6 ft tall, Martin may have presented more of a challenge than he imagined. Either way, he pulled up a chair and explained what post-operative confusion was, despite having very little understanding of it himself. 'If psychiatric nursing taught me anything it was the ability to bullshit with the best of them and we settled down for a good natter about his operation, life, job, family, ambitions, hopes and desires.'

Martin also confesses: I stayed with him for about half-an-hour to avoid having to go back to proper work. When a staff nurse eventually stuck her head apprehensively around the door, I was satisfied to see the surprise on her face that all was well, and felt not a little smug.

Bed making

The ritual of bed baths is only superseded by the ritual of 'how to make a bed'. This involved two nurses, one either side of the bed, working together to strip it and make it in perfect harmony, folding the blankets and sheets back into thirds and into the laundry skip or stored tidily on a bench or chair at the end of the bed. Laundry was never dropped on the floor. As one sister at Royal Infirmary Edinburgh, declared: 'Synchronisation of movement is the secret of good bed making.'

Every nurse remembers the precision of bedmaking – hospital corners and turning the top sheet down exactly so. In the US it took just one nurse to make a bed, but this never caught on in the UK where it was considered to be much quicker if two nurses danced the ritual. Hospital corners symmetrical, the pillow cases with the open edge facing away from the door and the wheels of the bed turned in and the bedside chair or stool always on the side of bed away from door. Some hospitals stipulated that each bed had to be made within three minutes. Dating back to Florence Nightingale and the Crimea, pillow cases opened away from the door so that dust did not blow into them. Wheels turned in was a safety precaution so that no one tripped over them.

There was often a hospital crest on the sheets or a stripe down the middle, with the name of the hospital embroidered into it, leading to a song and dance about the exact positioning of this. A stripe usually had to be absolutely central on the turned over top sheet – the turnover itself measuring exactly 18 inches. One nurse recalls: 'If a patient was in bed the stripe had to run straight down from their nose!'

At St Thomas's Hospital, one nursing sister carried a ruler and set square with her to ensure that the hospital crest was always displayed centrally 9 inches from the bottom of the bed and equidistant from the sides. The hospital corners had to be at precisely 45 degrees. On being challenged by a student nurse, muttering that it was impossible to get the dimensions so exact, the nursing sister marched the student to a bed and guided her through making it, demonstrating that it was perfectly possible. The patients in that four-bedded bay regaled everyone with the story for the next few days.

Susie remembers on one paediatric ward at St Bartholomew's Hospital:

> Sister Kenton used to insist that the cot counterpanes were
> turned at 3 o'clock, so all the teddy bears faced the opposite
> direction. Goodness knows why, and I certainly didn't dare
> to ask! I think it was just to give us something else to do at
> a time when God forbid there might be a few minutes lull.

Gone are the days of bed curtains needing to be taken down and washed as they are now disposable. In the 1920s, curtain washing was a four weekly routine – a practice that had long fallen by the wayside by the middle of the twentieth century and was hardly thought about unless there were obvious stains on them. Maybe infection control had slipped a little.

Ward cleaning on a Sunday remains a feature even today. David recalls while working in ITU, 'furiously cleaning things with a damp duster that were already clean'.

I certainly remember endless quiet Sundays spent gazing at shelves of spotless equipment in the treatment room or shining bedpans in the sluice, wondering just how much cleaning was good enough. Much later when I had a home of my own I would often consider the irony of being at work cleaning what was already clean when my own home hadn't seen any kind of dusting in months.

The purpose of weekend cleaning was as much to keep nurses busy than for any real need to clean. Dragging heavy laundry bags up corridors (any day of the week), washing bed pans and cleaning clinical rooms that were already clean was quite dispiriting. True, there are some things that really need checking and cleaning – the underside of commodes for instance– which is no great way to spend your Sunday.

In the 1960s, Linda says that during visiting hours (one hour a day in the afternoon), student nurses retired to the sluice to wash and polish the stainless steel with turpentine and stack it, all sparkling, on the racks and shelves. 'Nothing looks more beautiful than racks of brightly shining bedpans, bottles, bowls and sputum mugs.'

Earlier in the twentieth century, phenol lotion (also known as carbolic acid) was a powerful antiseptic usually measured at 5 per cent, or 1oz to 1 pint, and used for cleaning bedpans, urinals and other ward equipment.

Coloured pink, it was used as a preservative and disinfectant for ligatures, sutures and rubber tubing and was one of the many hazards that nurses had to be aware of because they were urged not to get it on their skin or the patient as it caused 'serious kidney disorganisation'.

Hazards

Nurses were at risk from all kinds of hazards that would not be tolerated now. The risk of scalding from sterilisers on the ward, boilers in theatre, or kettles in the kitchen was rife. From the 1960s the supply and maintenance of sterile equipment was taken from the wards and managed in a central sterile supply department (CSSD) giving nurses considerably less to do and reduced the risk of burns at work. Protests about the effect this would have on nurse training were overridden by what Monica Baly in *Nursing and Social Change*, describes as: 'alarming disclosures about cross infection.'

Despite this, sterilisers known as 'little sisters', still remained on surgical wards for small instruments to be handily sterilised in the treatment room.

Many theatres retained their own sterilising facility for a few years after that. Jan trained in the 1970s in Birmingham and remembers a room full of sterilisers in theatres. 'Once instruments were sterilised we took the trays out; I don't know how we didn't get burned.'

Others remember boilers in the main theatres and risking life and limb coiling the rubber suction tubing and tying it, making sure the lumen was full of water so that it sterilised inside and out. Extracting it from the boiler with Cheatles forceps and twirling the tubing round to empty it was quite an art, and you had to dance out of the way to avoid scalded feet.

Patients were also at risk. Hot air treatment was favoured at one time for the treatment of shock and collapse, for local rheumatoid conditions and also to induce excessive sweating which was thought to be good for kidney disease as it ensured the removal of waste products and was a 'general cleansing of the tissues'.

The procedure is described in 1940s *Modern Professional Nursing*. Hot water bottles were popped into the bed to warm the patient's feet and then all the blankets removed except one which was placed over a cradle the length of the body, with only the patient's head protruding, to create an 'air marquee'. Hot air was blown into this via a spirit lamp placed in a metal trayful of sand as protection against fire. Temperatures inside the tent could reach 140–175°F (60–80°C). Nurses were instructed not to leave the patient and to take their pulse and temperature every minute (which is difficult if separate readings are to be obtained) because a minute too long in the heat could mean, 'Much harm could be done to the human machinery, resulting in collapse, breathlessness, quick pulse, flushing and suffocation.'

Patients might remain in this hot tent for up to twenty minutes and then allowed to gradually cool down.

Burns are a serious and fairly regular feature for patients attending A&E today, but at one time they were very common due to poor living conditions. In the 1940s and 1950s, Mary remembers that it was quite usual for people not to have plumbed hot water and so they boiled water over fires for bathing, putting themselves and their families at all kinds of risk.

Other frequent but less scary hazards, particularly in old hospital buildings, are cockroaches and mice. At Bart's, turning on the light in the underground passageways and some of the theatres sent cockroaches scuttling for dark corners.

Ruby remembers being advised by night sister that one of the patients had given the ward some Nice biscuits which were in the kitchen. Disappointingly, Ruby found the biscuits a bit tough and a bit disgusting, not like usual Nice biscuits, so she only ate part of one. In the morning night sister came around and asked her if she had found the biscuits for the mice. Apparently, Ruby was supposed to put the specially poisoned biscuits out to trap the mice who appeared out of the heating pipes at night. She didn't let on that she had tried one and fortunately, she didn't come to any harm.

Eating and drinking

Millicent Ashdown records in her 1940s text that when nursing pneumonia, nourishing liquid is necessary until after the crisis – the term used for the sudden change for the better when recovery looks possible in conditions such as pneumonia, erysipelas (acute infection with a rash) or measles. She stipulates that such liquid should be given: '...in quantities of 5 oz every two hours – milk, egg flip, white coffee, fruit juice with glucose, milk Bovril. Regular feeding is most important...'.

On my first ward, I found myself being asked to make scrambled eggs for any number of patients. While it seemed acceptable to be green about what I regarded as nursing, I felt a little ashamed to admit to my lack of basic culinary skills, but I soon found that lots of my contemporaries were similarly ill-equipped. What had we been doing with our teenage years when we could have been learning to cook eggs?! In those days nurses often made snacks for patients who couldn't face the regular meals. It's not possible to provide this kind of comfort these days as any food in the ward kitchen is usually locked away to prevent anyone – nurse or patient – stealing it. It is also packaged and processed like aeroplane food and not at all appetising unlike freshly cooked eggs – even made by an amateur.

For a long time post war, when rationing was still in place, patients were allocated an egg box in the kitchen and eggs were brought in for them by relatives. Patients could then request boiled, poached, scrambled or fried, making the breakfast routine even more rushed and complex. Many a nurse admits she failed to get the right egg cooked in the right way to the right patient.

One tale lingers post war from Hill End hospital in St Albans, the hospital to which Bart's decamped during the Second World War. There was one nurse who, legend has it, skilfully cooked breakfast for a whole ward of patients on a single Bunsen burner. She would call out, 'boiled, fried or poached', remembers Vera, and we would put in the patient's order and she would produce a perfectly cooked egg.

It was in that meagre post-war period that Eunice says she was given an egg and un-scrubbed potatoes on night duty from which she was supposed to construct a meal for herself. She says they used arachis oil (usually used to rub on patients' legs to relieve dry skin) to fry them. Arachis oil, more commonly known now as peanut oil, might present all kinds of risk to those with allergy as is common these days.

Mary Anne recalls the routine of preparing breakfast for the patients at the end of night duty in the kitchens by the Nightingale wards. 'We had to cook a massive pot of porridge, boiled eggs and hot buttered toast for all 30 or so patients and make tea in huge teapots.'

Tea at the old Hackney hospital when I trained in the 1980s, was also made in huge teapots: milk and sugar already added. No need to ask!

The evening drinks trolley was a comforting routine for patients and nurses alike. It signalled the near end of the evening shift and those patients who had been in hospital too long were happy to take over the job, wheeling the trolley down the long wards, knowing each patient's 'usual', having a gentle chat. It was also a source of practical jokes. Eunice remembers 'losing' the drinks trolley on the male orthopaedic ward at Hill End only to discover the men had disguised it under bedclothes making it appear like one of the large bed cradles they used to keep blankets off broken limbs.

Other comforting routines included scones made by Sister Lawrence in the 1970s in the ward kitchen at Bart's. She kept a jug of milk in the kitchen cupboard so it would be sour for Sunday scone making. The junior nurse on duty would distribute these to all nursing officers and ward sisters working that weekend. It's not recorded whether more junior staff were also allowed to eat the scones.

Mild theft was an issue from time to time. When I trained, I liked snatching cups of cold milk out of the refrigerated 'cow' in the ward kitchen, while laying up the drinks trolley for the evening round. It was either that or the newly discovered alcohol while out partying that led to weight gain in my early twenties!

Eating the patient's leftover food is theft and an absolute no-no – at least for me. This is principle, but it helps that hospital food rarely looks appetising. It is easy to see why people do it, though. In today's hospitals, nurses hardly have time to pee let alone eat, canteens are open only for a few hours and do not provide the twenty-four hour service they once did, and staff have to make do with vending machines or expensive sandwiches from shops like Marks and Spencer that have taken over hospital reception areas. If the food is going to be thrown away, what harm is there in eating it? Of course, fundamentally, it is stealing and it could be classified as unprofessional, according to the Nursing and Midwifery Code of Conduct.

Chapter 10

Once the Dust has Settled

'Some of the remedies used verge on witchcraft… its origins in the mythology of nursing.'

I was always quite scared, in a 'Dr Who' kind of way, of the man on my first ward who used to pop out his false eye at night and put it in a pot on his locker. I was terrified I would inadvertently catch the eye looking at me while on night duty, or that he would ask me to pass it to him. We were supposed to help him take it out, but I reckoned that if he managed it at home then he could manage it in hospital and I used to give him a wide berth towards the end of a late shift when patients were settling down for the night. I never knew why he had a false eye; he probably had an interesting story to tell, but eyes, generally, made me feel a bit queasy and I was glad I didn't ever work on an ophthalmic ward or theatres.

A detached retina occurs when the thin layer at the back of the eye (retina) tears or becomes loose. It needs to be treated quickly to stop it permanently affecting sight. It is more common in older people when there is a change to the jelly like substance (vitreous humour) inside the eye.

These days, patients having retinal surgery are usually treated as day cases and they can rest at home. Contrast this to the complete bed rest that was required back in the 1940s. Aunt Molly remembers that it was vital to wait until the retina was fully repaired and during that time patients had to be nursed entirely flat. She recalls: 'They were not to move and they had to be washed and fed for a week, may be two weeks.'

The patients were usually elderly and were very often confused, probably never having been in hospital before. Quite often, says Molly, they would suddenly get out of bed and go charging down the ward. One such patient was an elderly and confused ex-nursing sister. Molly says: 'She was up and down with her head in the locker. We couldn't stop her. We were terrified of the trouble we would get into.'

It was containing the older gentlemen that was the real test. It's a universal fact that men are not bothered about anyone seeing them naked. Aunt Molly says that when the gentlemen got out of bed 'without permission', they never put their clothes on.

> You would see a gentleman stark naked get out of his bed
> and go into his locker and take out a small attaché case and
> go walking down the ward (as if) on his way home.

Hand in glove

There is much conjecture that the regular wearing of gloves came in when the global AIDS epidemic swept through the mid-1980s. Ignorance about how the condition was spread and the lack of treatment made people question (perhaps at long last) their infection-control practice. It may be fair to say that with the advent of antibiotics, we had all become a little too complacent about infection control and cleanliness. Florence would have been horrified.

Chief scrub nurse Caroline Hampton is regarded as the first person to wear rubber gloves in the operating theatre. She developed dermatitis from handling the disinfectants and as the chief of surgery at John Hopkins Hospital, USA, William Halstead, found her to be an 'unusually efficient woman', he set about finding a solution. The Goodyear Rubber Company developed some rubber gloves that proved so successful that others in the operating room began to use them too and they were first used in surgery in 1894. It also led to romance and Caroline Hampton and Halstead were married a year later.

At first Halstead did not use gloves himself. They were used by nurses and assistants but rarely by the doctors (except for the open bone and joint operations). It was only when Dr Joseph Bloodgood, Halsted's protege, wore gloves during surgery and published a report on over 450 hernia operations with a near 100 per cent drop in the infection rate by using gloves, that Halstead also started wearing them. Up until then, the gloves had perhaps been perceived as there to protect the wearer and not the patient. Arguably an attitude that has crept back in now that gloves are routinely worn for almost every procedure and task.

Wearing gloves for anything other than sterile procedures or the messiest of episodes involving bodily fluids took a long time to translate onto the wards. One former professor of nursing, says: 'We were told it was humiliating to the patient to put gloves on. You were making the patient feel untouchable.'

Consequently, a 'no touch' technique was necessary for dressing wounds. Mary's 1940's nursing text book, *Modern Professional Nursing* says, quite sternly: 'The "no touch" technique which was talked of so much during World War II is not by any means new: it has been in existence many years and is very simple and easy.'

The 'no touch' or 'aseptic' technique continued to be applied for generations after, and while it wasn't necessarily simple or easy, it was something you learned. The method involved using forceps or tweezers to clean wounds and apply dressings. Once grasped it was fiddly to unlearn: not unlike moving from a gearstick car to an automatic. When I did a return to practice course in 2002, gloves were the norm and forceps considered unnecessary, yet it felt clumsy and wrong to be touching anything with my (gloved) hands.

Successfully changing a dressing using the aseptic technique while under the watchful gaze of a clinical nurse tutor was one of the more nerve wracking of the four practical assessments a student nurse had to perform. Gail remembers: 'My aseptic technique assessment was to shorten a corrugated drain – I bet nobody would consider not using gloves for something like that any more.'

Wounds have drains inserted to draw out pus and excess fluid and they can be fiddly to manage. There is some controversy as to whether drains are even that useful as they may increase the risk of infection. The use of drains is often based on what the surgeon prefers or has always used. Gail says:

> At some point gloves started to appear in dressing packs – I don't remember when. We had a SHO (senior house officer) in A&E once who refused to wear gloves for anything – and it never caused any problems. That must have been in the early 1980s.

These days, boxes of gloves are always to hand and patients expect you to wear them. The pendulum may be swinging back the other way as people point out that staff do not always wear gloves appropriately. For instance, putting on gloves at the beginning of a shift and working through numerous jobs is about self-protection rather than preventing the spread of infection.

In the early days, rubber gloves were cleaned for reuse. Nurses would soak the gloves in cold water to get rid of any blood or discharge and then wash them in warm soapy water until clean. They were then rinsed and hung up to dry; later to be turned inside out to dry on the inside. They were examined for holes and if necessary, repaired with a small piece of rubber cut from a discarded glove and mended in the same way as mending a bicycle tube. The skills required of nurses! Gloves to be sterilised were placed in pairs into the dressing drums and sent to be autoclaved.

Sterilising of instruments was done on the ward certainly until the 1960s, may be later in some places, when they started to be replaced by central sterile supply departments (CSSDs). The length of boiling varied hugely over the years from twenty minutes for some instruments to two minutes. Invariably instruments would then be soaked in Lysol.

Lysol is a disinfectant still found today in various cleaning products. It has a strong odour and many a nurse remembers using it for cleaning on the wards with repercussions for unprotected hands.

Wound care and dressings

Often the ward routine was based on long-forgotten evidence. Nurses who trained in the 1930s and 40s were taught that wound dressings were done when there were no visitors present and at least an hour after the morning cleaning had been completed: once the dust had settled. Dust was considered a potential risk to wound healing. This allowed for time to perform often complicated dressings in a calm, clean atmosphere, protecting the patient. Such routines made sense in a world where cleanliness was almost the only combatant against infection. They were still routine when I trained in the 1980s and beyond.

In the 1930s and 40s, dry wound dressing and swabs were prepared by nurses, usually while on night duty, and placed in a drum and sent away to be autoclaved.

The dressing round was done in order from the cleanest to the dirtiest wound. In this task orientated world, a staff nurse with a probationer (student nurse) would go around the ward and dress the wounds. The beauty of this was that with staff likely to be working six days a week, the same person could see any improvement or deterioration in the wound.

During the round each fresh dressing would be taken out of the drum as the nurses went from patient to patient. So, what was initially sterile was no longer sterile once the drum was opened. The drums were packed in an ordered way so that what was taken out first was needed first, whether swabs or theatre gowns. This is the kind of organisation that is second nature to nurses of a certain era.

Preparing a dressing trolley didn't change much between the 1940s to the 1980s. Clean the trolley, sterile dressing and assorted equipment on the top shelf, additional bandages on the lower shelf. Except in the 1980s, the dressing packs came from CSSD all neatly packaged while in the 1940s nurses sterilised the instruments themselves on the ward and made up the dressings. At that time, nurse and patient were each required to wear a mask while the dressing was done – and it was advised that there be two nurses present for each dressing. In the 1930s and 1940s masks were not disposable but required laundering, which was done on the ward, adding to the burden of nursing tasks.

The cleaning of the trolley was itself a ritual and, while clean is important, it is questionable just how often it needed to be cleaned given that only a sterile dressing pack had been placed on the top with accessories on the lower shelf – all dirty dressings were disposed of in the attached paper bag. Still we cleaned. A spritz of ubiquitous Sudol and a wipe with paper towels.

Trolleys, originally called dressing wagons, were part of the ritual, as Sarah remembers from her time at what was the London Hospital:

> The dressing trolley was sacrosanct, properly cleaned every time and items placed on the appropriate shelf and each dressing had a particular procedure depending on the wound or operation that had been carried out. We had to name all instruments and dressings on the trolley.

Wound healing is a complex process and over the years there have been myriad approaches and techniques to encourage healing and prevent infection. Nurses of every generation have been irritated by a ritual requested by many surgeons – that was to take down a dressing prior to a ward round. Removing the dressing sometimes pulled away healing tissue and exposing the wound to the air did not improve the rate of healing. Diana worked with a ward sister at the RIE who insisted that dressings be left untouched and that if there was a problem, she would inform the surgeon.

As Mike Walsh and Pauline Ford point out in their 1989 book *Nursing Rituals, research and rational actions*: 'Ritual and tradition are not the sole prerogative of nurses.'

They also note: 'Some of the remedies used verge on witchcraft... [and] has its origins in the mythology of nursing.'

Leeches and maggots

Leeches and maggots might fall into the category of 'witchcraft'. Carol trained in the early 1970s and was incredulous when she was sent down to pharmacy to collect leeches to use on wounds. She says: 'We rather giggled and thought it very dated.'

Leeches are used to relieve an area congested with blood by sucking it up. They can be applied to those undergoing plastic surgery or who are at risk of losing a limb due to the side effects of diabetes. They can also be used to treat blood clots, varicose veins and dangerously high blood pressure. Medicinal leeches have three jaws with tiny rows of teeth. They pierce a person's skin with their teeth and insert Hirudin, a substance that prevents blood clotting. Carol acknowledges their modern-day usage:

> Recently my friend's leg was saved by the use of leeches to debride a nasty wound. No popping down to pharmacy and collecting them in a pot after they had been removed from a tank. The modern leeches come especially bred, sanitised and cost a walloping £1,000 per batch.

Carol also reports of another incident where a huge haematoma (blood clot) threatened the success of a mastectomy operation. 'Emergency batches of leeches were ferried by police escort to the hospital and the leeches did their job.'

111

The leeches are left on the skin to extract blood for twenty to forty-five minutes at a time. According to Ann Lamb's notes in 1932: 'the average leech will draw off 1 oz of blood'.

Ann notes that the skin must be clean but free from soap. A drop of milk may be dropped over the part to be treated and nurses must watch that the leech does not wander, having taken the precaution to 'plug all adjoining cavities!'

Modern Professional Nursing warns that a leech has to be: 'humoured before he will consent to perform...'.

This includes ensuring the patient's clean skin has no strong scent of perfume or disinfectant and that the patient can't feel the leeches: 'The area is covered by a piece of lint in which holes are cut to allow the leech to bite: slimy parasites such as this should never be felt by the patient.'

Indeed, it advises that nervous patients might need to be blindfolded.

Thelma qualified in 1978 and worked as a staff nurse for six months on Observation Ward at St Bartholomew's Hospital. She recounts:

> We had a tank of three leeches on the ward. Sister Harvey showed us how to clean the area that the leech was to be applied to and then paint a milk and sugar solution so that the leech would bite on. After the leech had drunk its fill and fallen off you had to roll it in salt so that it would vomit – if you didn't, they wouldn't feed for ages.

Thelma says the method was very successful for an elderly lady who had a swollen black eye and the swelling was reduced enough for a detached retina to be discovered and treated. It was less successful on a medical student referred one Saturday afternoon with a badly swollen and bruised ear. Leeches were prescribed to hopefully avoid the 'cauliflower' type ear that used to be common among rugby players. Thelma says:

> I wasn't too keen on handling the leech and used a kitchen spoon. Needless to say, the leech rolled off down his shirt collar and he was dancing around terrified that the leech would attach elsewhere! We managed in the end but it wasn't that successful and years later when we worked together, I saw he had a fat ear.

Cate reports leeches being effectively used to bring down someone's dangerously high blood pressure, while my sister in law recounts the story of A&E staff working out how to unlatch a pet leech attached to her brother, a medieval history enthusiast who kept the leeches for when he was being a physician in re-enactments. He had let one of his leeches have a feed and couldn't then remove it.

Using maggots to clean wounds dates back centuries with each generation discovering their powers, particularly in wartime when soldiers with wounds infested with maggots did better than those that didn't. The introduction of penicillin around the time of the Second World War meant that maggot therapy generally dropped out of fashion.

There is a bit of a psychological clash between keeping a wound clean and our association of maggots with dirt. Pat used them in the burns unit at Glasgow Royal Infirmary and says: 'They made us feel creepy and once the burn dressings were finished, we were allowed to go change our uniforms.'

Gail was castigated as a student nurse for helping a homeless man to wash, cleaning all the maggots out of his wound as she did so. They were in fact helping to heal the wound, even if they hadn't been put there deliberately.

Maggots are still sometimes used for wounds that just won't heal. Research has shown that their secretions contain an enzyme which can kill bacteria because they disinfect as they work and they also stimulate the development of healthy tissues.

More weird and wonderful techniques

Cupping is described as an ancient therapy used originally as part of a ritual to rid the body of evil spirits. Over the twentieth century and earlier, 'wet cupping' was used as an 'artificial method of leeching' or bloodletting, while 'dry cupping' was used to encourage blood and other fluids to the skin's surface. According to *Modern Nursing*, a tray of twelve cupping glasses is set out with Vaseline, methylated spirit, sterilised blotting paper and matches.

> Vaseline is carefully applied to the edges of the cupping
> glasses and a small piece of blotting paper, saturated with

methylated spirit, is placed inside the cup. The paper is set alight and immediately the glass is pressed firmly over the area to be treated. The burning of the paper goes on for a moment while the air lasts, then a vacuum is created and the skin is drawn up into the glass, holding in position firmly.

Apparently, if cupping glasses are not available a wine glass is a good substitute. In the late 1940s, a more modern type of cup came into use called a 'Bier's suction apparatus', which consisted of a glass bell connected to a rubber tube and a hand suction pump. As the air was pumped out of the bell it sucked in the tissue, drawing the pus out of a carbuncle.

A modern take on cupping came into public consciousness when it was talked about during the 2016 Rio Olympics as a method of relieving muscle tension. Some of the swimmers could be seen with round cup marks on their backs.

Lotions and potions

There was a range of wound-cleaning methods to choose from – some effective, a few discredited. Chief among these is EUSOL – Edinburgh University Solution of Lime (an antiseptic solution prepared from chlorinated lime and boric acid). It was used to remove foreign material and cleanse the wound (debridement), remove dead tissue and pus (desloughing), and prevent and control infection by antibacterial action (disinfection).

Nurses used to tip it into an open wound and watch it fizz. It made dressings fun and gave all the appearance of thoroughly cleaning the wound. However, the harm it caused as a skin irritant, its destruction of healthy tissue, and slow wound healing, and even that it might cause cancer, came to be realised and it was withdrawn from use.

Women who had vulval cancer were treated surgically with a vulvectomy (removal of the vulva) and required what one nurse described as 'hideous' daily dressings which included cleaning with hydrogen peroxide. That must have really stung. This surgery is much better now and the skin does not break down so frequently. Honey was also used to help the wounds heal. For example, for ano-vagional fistulas, where a tract has opened up between the anus and the vagina, allowing faecal material to pass through the vagina (most commonly caused by injury during childbirth), were treated by cleaning every few hours with hydrogen peroxide and then packed with honey and ribbon gauze.

Honey is a proven wound-healing success. Effective on burns, surgical wounds, venous leg ulcers, pressure sores, and even the extreme condition of necrotising fasciitis, honey seems to have a cleaning effect on the wound and keeps it moist, so allowing tissue to revitalise. It's thought to have antibacterial and anti-inflammatory effects. Sarah used honey tulle (open weave gauze impregnated with honey) in tins, as a district nurse in the 1980s. Liz recalls honey and onion dressings from her days working as a district nurse. They were the idea of the patient who swore by them as they had been used in her family for generations. Liz says she's not sure if it was the honey or the onion that worked but the dressing kept the wound clean and the patient found it comfortable and declined all other treatment options.

These days, medical-grade honey is used – a specifically manufactured product that is sterilised to remove impurities and any potential bacteria. It is used on all manner of wounds – from caesarean sections to diabetic foot ulcers. It has also been used to kickstart healing in wounds that have been resistant to antibiotics.

Mercurochrome, which dyes the skin a chemical orange-red was popular for much of the twentieth century as an antiseptic for abrasions and minor wounds. It is still available today although banned in many countries such as the US, Switzerland, Brazil, France and Germany because it contains mercury.

Making poultices

Kaolin poultices were made of methyl salicylate, glycerine, thymol and aromatic oil wrapped in lint and gauze and were used to draw out infection from a wound. Mary says that when she was working in A&E in the early 1950s, the nurses made up a kaolin poultice each morning, from a square of sheeting, filled with kaolin. It was rolled up tightly and put behind the steriliser to keep warm.

A section was cut off from the warm kaolin roll whenever it was needed. Heat was considered an essential feature of the poultice and nurses were urged to remove the old one quickly and apply the new one at once so that the area did not have time to cool. Undoubtedly, heat is soothing for pain and helps to draw out infection but keeping a poultice warm all day behind a steriliser sounds like a perfect breeding ground for infection.

Barbara recalls in *Sisters, memories from the courageous nurses of World War Two*:

> We had to loosen the lid of the kaolin tin, then put it in an old enamel pan part-filled with water then put it to boil. I cannot remember what it boiled on. I know that I won't be the only nurse to have forgotten about it and returned to find the pan had gone dry. Then we made a sort of sandwich of four inch gauze pads and the kaolin paste was the filling. There was some kind of old knife to spread the paste. The tin was by now very hot, wet and slippery. Quite a triumph to appear through the sluice door carrying it between two enamel plates to your grateful patient.

According to 1923 records from the Royal Infirmary Edinburgh, crushed linseed was often used for a poultice. Linseed contains oil which is useful both as an emollient and to retain heat, which can draw out infection. The RIE record how to make this poultice. The nurse had to half fill a basin with boiling water, then quickly sprinkle in the linseed while stirring with a spatula. When the mixture came clean away from the edge of the basin, the nurse would turn it out on a piece of linen and spread it evenly and quickly with the spatula, dipping the spatula in hot water between each stroke. The linseed meal was spread to a depth of about 1.4 inches and rolled up.

Sphagnum moss, used on a large scale in the First World War, was still being used to dress wounds into the 1940s. The moss could be found throughout the UK and so was a cheaper alternative to cotton for dressings which had been commandeered for making uniforms and the manufacture of munitions. The moss was thought able to absorb up to twenty times its volume in liquid, and could restrict bacterial growth due to its acidity, and antiseptic properties. It was used on a smaller scale during the Second World War and in 1940, requests for sphagnum moss were advertised in the press, with 250 Red Cross workers in Glasgow working to process the moss that volunteers collected. The moss was then sorted, dried, and packed into muslin bags and used as dressings.

Rolling bandages and making dressings including Gamgee tissue was still an important feature of a post-war nurse's work. Pioneered by Sam Gamgee in the 1840s, the Gamgee dressing was a sandwich of gauze with a cotton-wool filling to make a dry absorbent dressing – similar to many sterile dressings that are now manufactured.

Before the introduction of hospital sterile supply departments, making up dressings and rolling bandages were standard nursing duties but the practice of making dressings continued for generations afterwards.

Sarah trained at Bradford School of Nursing and remembers a placement at an orthopaedic hospital in 1984:

> We used to sew our own traction kits, using rolls of Elastoplast with thick lengths of wick attached. These were sewn by hand (ouch), no thimble, using strong thread. When a patient had traction applied one part of the roll was used then a new piece of wick applied for the next patient…This was part of the weekend work usually sewn as we sat in the middle of the ward during Sunday visiting.

As Sarah says, this didn't take into account any of the infection-control rules of single use per patient, that is part of modern day practice.

Many-tailed bandages, made of a long vertical strip with four strips of bandages coming off it horizontally, were used to support wounds after major abdominal surgery. Sue remembers making the bandages, stitching the tails to the vertical panel. No wonder nursing schools wanted to know about applicants' needlework skills!

In Mary's day, it was common to learn nursing rituals 'off by heart', which nearly seventy years later she could still quote:

> R is for roll the bandage we love
> Start inside to outside
> Below to above

At the Brook Hospital in London in 1988, Alison worked with a ward sister who she describes as having the 'poise and deportment of a finishing school graduate', while also being something of a 'demon bandager', having undertaken her orthopaedic nursing course in the late 1950s. The sister taught the students how to bandage: barrel of the bandage with the open end uppermost in the hand, regular (three-quarters of an inch, maybe) overlapping layers up the arm and secured on the outer surface, where one could see the safety pin and also where it wouldn't press into any part of the patient's body.

Chapter 11

Theatre Theatricals

'It was impossible for me to walk across the floor of theatre without
tripping over a piece of equipment, contaminating the
sterile field, or knocking over a tray of instruments.'

Operating theatres are the home of drama. Some of it manufactured in
order to stroke the egos of surgeons, but mostly it is the sheer heroics of
life-saving operations that hold their rightful ground-breaking place. The
twentieth century saw the advent of organ transplants, the routinisation
of once cutting-edge heart and brain surgery, the successful separation
of conjoined twins and huge leaps in spinal surgery and trauma repair.

Motorcyclists, along with horse riders and pedal cyclists, are still the
most likely road users to end up in A&E needing urgent surgery. But
in the 1940s, Mary remembers the frequency and seriousness of them.
People didn't wear helmets, and often the injuries were to girls riding
pillion with their boyfriends and falling off the back of the motorbikes.
Mary says: 'The thing that made the biggest difference was when we
learned to immobilise the head after an accident.'

Wearing a crash hat on a motorbike did not become compulsory until
almost thirty years later in 1973.

If theatres are the home of drama, they are also home to boring rituals
that are essential to keeping patients safe and instruments sterile. There
is endless checking and rechecking and stocking of supplies, not to
mention cleaning, swab counting and sterilising. All of which I found
very dull and I discovered I was more squeamish than I had hoped –
disliking the gristly sounds of ear, nose and throat surgery and being
frankly horrified at the carpentry and sheer brutality of orthopaedic
surgery. This can be summed up in one nurse's experience observing a
total hip replacement: 'The consultant suddenly threw a hard lump of

bloody, increasingly hot cement at me and told me to knead it until it was hard! And I wasn't wearing gloves.'

Generally, as a nursing student, you were ignored in theatres unless a particularly menial job needed doing or someone more senior decided that you were to be the focus of entertainment.

Mary Anne says as a young student, she was the assisting scrub nurse on a urology list, during one of the first penile implants in the UK.

> The senior registrar assisting the consultant thought it would be funny to get me to hold the dish under the penis and made lots of comments about needing to get closer and it wouldn't bite me, that I needed to get used to handling these things. Everyone thought it was hilarious except me, who felt mortified!

Many rituals in theatres were the result of the superstitions of those who perform life-saving surgery on a daily basis – things as simple as the colour and design of scrubs, net hats and theatre clogs.

Dianne who worked in theatres in the 1960s and 1970s remembers:

> The laying up of instrument trolleys was to a strict system, determined by the type of operation. Packs were prepared in the sterile supply department, labelled, autoclaved and available for use as required, the instruments were autoclaved in the operating department and taken to a trolley covered with a sterilised cloth.
>
> All instruments and swabs were counted before the first incision, numbers recorded on a white board and all re-counted and accounted for before final closure of the wound.

Alison who worked in theatres in the same era says:

> After each operation the scrub nurse washed all the instruments under running water with a bristle brush – in what was called the 'dirty side'.
>
> Articles that could not be immersed in water were sterilised by formaldehyde in what we called a Porge. This was a steel cabinet with drawers and formaldeyde was in

the lowest tray – the Porge was turned on for several hours – and sterilisation was complete!

Endoscopes were sterilized in the dreaded CIDEX! Ghastly stuff with a ghastly smell.

Just as Menzies Lyth argued that routine on the wards was depersonalising, so Katz (1981) argues that the strict sterility and checking procedures employed in the operating room help to diffuse emotions and enable theatre staff to 'disconnect' with everyday life. If they did not, they would not be able to cope with the strangeness of seeing an unconscious person cut open or handling their organs and secretions. In this way, ritual contributes to the efficiency in theatre as everyone has a role to play focused on the goal of successful surgery.

Dianne says that some surgeons had specific requirements in relation to instruments. For example, an orthopaedic surgeon who used a 'domestic' screwdriver because it was comfortable in his hand. The plastic handle would not withstand autoclaving, so it was sterilised in solution. Others had favourite forceps and could become very angry if handed a different but more usual instrument for the procedure.

Alison says that in the 1960s consultants were treated with reverence and respect. Each had a book of exactly what *they* used for each operation and the theatre staff were to make sure every request was met. Senior Registrars pushed to have a book too – it was a signal that they had arrived!

Working at speed seems to be common among surgeons. One worked so quickly that she was renowned for collecting patients from the ward herself. And for another, Dianne remembers: '[He] operated very quickly and always left theatre rapidly. A student was positioned ready to undo his gown as he was walking away, should the gown not be undone as he reached the door, it would be torn off.'

The need to work as a team, reacting swiftly often in unspoken unity means that camaraderie between theatre staff is common but in such an intense atmosphere with some big egos, so are disagreements. Arguments about the music to be played during operations were rife in one theatre when I was a student with the surgeon demanding one thing and the anaesthetist changing it or turning if off mid-operation.

In another, one of the anaesthetists spent his time on the phone (in the days when phones were mounted on the wall outside the operating theatre and not handily in your pocket) having loud conversations about fast cars. He would toss a casual command to one of the operating department assistants (ODAs) or to a nurse, to 'mind the anaesthetic machine'. He was vaguely astonished when a nurse refused this request.

Reverence aside, Alison is clear that nurses lead the team in theatre. They are the patients' advocate and ensure that he is cared for to a high standard and that the surgical team undertaking the procedures has the best possible service.

At the curator's

At one time, before disposable equipment became the norm, instruments had to be repaired and serviced. Jean says: 'The curator was the servicer and repairer of a lot of hospital equipment, repairing instruments, issuing new glass syringes, sharpening needles, lending out unusual things requested by wards.'

The expression 'at the curator's or 'doing the round', as in 'gone to see the curator', could be a coded message. At weekends, if it was quiet, the senior staff might go off duty, telling their junior that if anyone called the message was that they had gone to the curator's. The caller would know, even if the student didn't, that, barring an emergency, they wouldn't be back in that day.

Ginny had nursed the curator on her first ward and this always stood her in good stead when she needed an instrument fixed. It also made her popular with theatre staff who asked her to run this errand.

One theatre sister's announcement of a trip to the curator's could actually mean a visit to the bank which was not to the little branch of National Westminster just across the hospital square, but to Coutts in Sloane Square sometimes via the cobbler and picture framer. That was when she had not delegated the task to a student or staff nurse, saying: 'take your time'.

As a nursing student you only survived in theatres if you grasped the routine and saw where you could fit in. You avoided the arguments going on over your head by keeping busy in stock cupboards or linen stores. Little was really explained; you had to absorb it by osmosis. For those who were clumsy or lacking in confidence, it could be nerve wracking. Linda remembers: 'It was impossible for me to walk across the floor of theatre without tripping over a piece of equipment, contaminating the sterile field, or knocking over a tray of instruments.'

The scene was set therefore for what Linda describes as 'her finest hour'. She was standing as directed by the theatre sister in a particular floor square when sister beckoned her over and whispered in her ear so no one else could hear: 'There's a swab missing, find it … on the floor.'

Linda, amazed at being allocated such an important task, got down on her hands and knees, crawling around the theatre and under the operating table. She realised that suddenly there was a deathly silence, her eyes were in line with a large pair of green theatre boots and she looked up into the surgeon's face as he looked down at her. He had stopped the operation and all eyes were on her, surgeon, registrar, houseman, anaesthetist, nursing staff. He asked: 'Well, well nurse, are you having a pleasant time down there?'

Crimson-faced, Linda began to stand up, directly under the instrument tray, whereupon sister yelled at her to stop, to get down and not to dare touch anything.

Linda crawled away on her hands and knees out of the theatre to the back room, laughter ringing in her ears.

Jane was less intimidated. She trained at King's College in the 1980s along with her future husband who records their experiences in *The New Nightingale Chronicles*. During one long operating list, the theatre was a mass of green drapes and packed with medical and nursing students observing the operation.

Jane, leaning rather bored against the wall of the theatre, was startled into action by the theatre sister barking at her to fetch an additional instrument pack. Unsure how to pass it across the crowded theatre without contaminating the operating field, Jane took firm hold of the heavy metal tray, tightly wrapped and taped, and lobbed it over the oblivious patient, past the startled surgeon and toward the scrubbed sister, who, to her credit, leapt into the air and caught the instrument tray in full flight. This met with cheers from the watching medical students: ''Ows that!'

Even the anaesthetist looked up from his crossword to exclaim: 'Oh well caught old girl.'

Jane later claimed that the ensuing uproar and warning she received were quite disproportionate as she felt her actions at the time were logical. It certainly became the stuff of legend at King's.

Of course, a bunch of medical students is not always so brave. Alison recalls a so-called 'dirty' case – left to the end of the list. It was a debridement of a diabetic foot. Those who have diabetes are at risk of what is called diabetic neuropathy, where they have poor sensation and don't feel pain from injury or damage to their legs and feet. As a consequence, they can develop quite serious ulcers and ultimately may face amputation. Alison says the man's foot was very bad, with necrotic blackish toes hanging by threads:

> The surgeon pared away like a chiropodist on speed and as the metatarsals appeared like white webbing in the slough the semicircle of avidly observing medical students began to sway. One by one, starting with the biggest, they toppled and swooned.

At the sister's and surgeon's bidding, the student nurses grabbed a foot each and dragged away the bodies:

> We propped them up against the wall once they began to regain colour and consciousness and then went round with vomit bowls and cups of sweet tea, depending on the need.

Back from theatre

Post operatively, nurses care for patients in what is called 'recovery' usually close to the operating theatre, monitoring their vital signs and pain relief and caring for their breathing until they are conscious and no longer need a plastic airway. Ward nurses will then come and collect their charges. Eunice trained in the early 1950s. 'There was no recovery [area] in those days. When people came back from theatre, they came back [to the ward] with their airways in place.'

In preparation for a patient's return, the nurse would have ready a pewter vomit bowl, wooden bed-blocks to go under the end of the bed to combat any post-operative low blood pressure, which would be checked half hourly. Eunice says: 'We also had curved tongs to hand ready to grab the tongue if they swallowed it. We never received full instruction on how to use them but thankfully, I never had to!'

'Doing the obs' is a well-rehearsed ritual. Essential when a patient returns from theatre and usually done every fifteen minutes then every half hour, gradually reducing as the patient becomes more alert. All too often doing the obs was a task for a junior nurse and she may have been sent to do it just because she looked momentarily idle or perhaps the ward just did obs every four hours or twice daily until patients were discharged.

The accuracy of the observations was another issue. A junior or student might not be that efficient and, if afraid to ask, might not report anything out of the ordinary or might just think she has made a mistake. Counting respirations is quite a skill and invariably as soon as you glance at a patient's chest to count how often it rises and falls, the patient will speak to you throwing your counting out. As Mike Walsh and Pauline Ford comment, more than one consultant has been heard to say wryly: 'It is remarkable that every patient on this ward has a respiratory rate of 20!'

Preoperative preparations

The preoperative rituals start before the patient reaches the theatre doors. Again, these are mostly for safety reasons – checking that patient and operation details are correct. This checking and rechecking are becoming a modern ritual. While it's vital for checks to be made, the risk is familiarity and complacency that a subsequent check will be done by someone else so subconsciously you may not give it your full attention.

In the past there were a few rituals which we hung onto and perhaps overplayed, admitting patients one or two days before surgery to make sure we had time to perform them all. There were bloods to be taken, sometimes a preoperative shave, almost certainly an enema or two glycerine suppositories in order to empty the bowel. Joy recalls: Our minor surgery [patients] came in sometimes two nights prior to surgery. The D&C [dilation and curettage] patients even had to have a vulval trim and two glycerine suppositories!

Sometimes, whisper it, early admission was a way of ensuring your patient had a bed and the operation for which they might have been waiting months, went ahead. These days, such manipulation of beds is outside the control of the ward manager or indeed the surgeon, and is closely controlled by bed managers who have oversight of the whole hospital.

The traditional shave as part of preop preparation was a 'ritual based on a myth,' according to Mike Walsh and Pauline Ford in their book *Nursing Rituals, Research and Rational Actions*. The original reason for a shave was to reduce the risk of infection when a surgical incision was made. However, apart from the embarrassment to all parties because the shave is usually in an intimate area of the body, there is a risk that it will cause cuts or abrasions which are themselves a source of infection. Judy, says:

> If your patient was having surgery 'down below', you approached them with a Bic razor and talcum powder in the vain hope they would shave themselves. Fortunately, most did but I remember quite early on in my training one patient refused, telling me he had never shaved down there before. Unbeknown to him, neither had I, so I cracked on, thinking, 'if my Dad could see me now'. I can only imagine the shaving rash that developed later.

Patients need to starve before going to theatre to ensure they won't vomit and inhale the content into their lungs when they are under anaesthetic.

Research has shown that four hours is the optimum time for which someone needs to starve before an operation, a rule that was in place in the 1940s with the advice that Bovril, glucose or lemonade could be given in small quantities up to two hours before operation.

The four hours is mostly observed today with nothing after that except a sip of water in order to take any premedication prescribed by the anaesthetist. However, at one time the requirement for patients to be nil by mouth (NBM) before surgery grew into a slightly out of control ritual. Starving patients from midnight for those on a morning theatre list was usual. While the list may have started at 09.00, it would go on until 13.00 or later so some patients would go hungry for longer than others.

It was not so much that nurses were unthinking about their patients, but that the unpredictable nature of surgery and, let's be honest, surgeons, meant that the order of a theatre list could change at any time. So, delaying when a patient first becomes 'nil by mouth' because they are last on the morning list can go wrong if the surgeon decides to put them first. Cases get postponed, which risks a patient being starved for double the amount of time, or cases get cancelled and people are brought to the front of the queue.

The other reason why a standard order of NBM from midnight went out was because of the sheer busyness of a ward at night. One set time for making everyone NBM meant less room for error. A NBM notice was duly hung above the patient's bed. Such notices have mostly been done away with, along with other signs depicting that a patient is hard of hearing or has impaired eyesight.

While patients may be starved for too long, the reverse also happens; I remember working in a day-case unit and admitting a patient for an afternoon procedure and he cheerfully admitted he had eaten a cheese sandwich and a cup of tea for his lunch not half an hour before. He was annoyed to hear that he would have to come back another day for his procedure. 'Not eating' means different things to different people.

Pre-theatre pregnancy tests were often done ritually without much thought as to a woman's age or medical history – clearly those who were post-menopausal or had been sterilised were not going to be pregnant. Yet, 'just to be sure', tests were often still done – the risk of operating on a woman who was found to be pregnant was too ghastly to contemplate. I thought this ritual had died with nurses being able to make a professional judgement as to its necessity, only to witness its resurrection very recently. As well as being an unnecessary ritual, it hints at women (still) not being trusted to know their own bodies.

Removing jewellery and cleaning off make up and nail polish are two other rituals that are still important before surgery. Electricity can travel to any metal on the body and so removing jewellery is to prevent patients being burned from the current that comes from the electrocautery unit. However, wedding rings are the exception. This is recognition of the ritual they play in our western culture. It is surely a myth that your marriage will end if you remove your wedding ring, but it is a deeply ingrained belief. The other reason of course is that many people cannot get their wedding rings off, their fingers having grown a little too plump over the years. For this reason, tape is applied over the ring.

Hospital staff are also banned from wearing jewellery, including wrist watches. The latter has long been the case for nurses who wear a fob watch, the custom for which originated from avoiding scratching a patient with it when caring for them. It also frees up nurses' hands as it can be read upside down. Wearing a fob watch is synonymous with nursing and, given the passing of hats, aprons, badges and buckles, one that is held onto by nurses everywhere.

Many staff continue to wear wedding rings. Studies have shown that while ring fingers carry more bacteria than one's other fingers, the kind of surgical scrubbing that is done before an operation removes bacteria to a significant extent. Also, while gloves may not provide total protection, they do provide a vital barrier.

Removing a patient's nail polish and makeup preoperatively is essential in order to observe any changes in a patient's skin colour during surgery. A pulse oximeter is attached to a patient's finger in order to measure oxygen levels. Nail polish or indeed acrylic nails may hinder this. People today are asked to remove at least two acrylic nails (one from each hand) so the pulse oximeter can be applied.

At one time, in the early part of the twentieth century, patients were required to have their heads covered when going to theatre – that is all women, and men who were bald. This would be a head shawl or linen cap. Out of this ritual came a notable artefact at the London hospital – a headscarf worn by those nurses who were operated on by a Mr James Sherren. The scarf was embroidered with their initials and was, until recently, on display at the Royal London Hospital.

Fashions in drugs given as premedication before surgery come and go almost as frequently as the anaesthetist who decides the regime, but for a long time in the 1970s and 1980s, intramuscular injections of Omnopom and Scopolamine were the ritual. Gail says: 'We gave "Om & Scop" as a pre-med and used to get told off by theatre staff if the pre-med was given too late or too soon.'

Getting the timing right was something of an art form – guessing when the surgeon was likely to be finishing the previous case, taking a judgement call from theatre staff on the timing in order to weigh up the optimum moment for the pre-med for the next patient.

Pain relief post-surgery consisted mostly of intramuscular injections of pethidine or morphine which nurses could give. Registered nurses now give intravenous pain relief or antiemetics if the patient is feeling nauseous, where once they had to wait for a doctor to do it. The patient can also now manage their own pain relief through the use of patient controlled analgesia (PCAs). At the click of a button the patient can discharge a controlled amount of analgesia to themselves via an intravenous syringe driver. As a result, giving intramuscular injections is a rarity these days.

Of course, as we all know, student nurses practised giving injections into oranges. My mother learnt via this method in the 1950s as I did in the 1980s. She with glass syringes, me with plastic and disposable.

I would argue that the training for this is more thorough today, although the experience on the ward is less frequent. Louise says that she and her fellow students are given a list of reading and virtual learning (quizzes and interactive websites) to do on injections, followed by two days learning about the different kinds of injections, and then practice giving them on mannequins. The good thing about the mannequin is that it's easier to talk to it like a human (unlike an orange!) but to be honest, Louise says, it still doesn't feel the same as injecting a human being.

Surgical nursing sees a rapid throughput of patients as they come in for surgery and go out again, especially these days when patients are admitted on the day of their operation, fingers and toes crossed that it will still go ahead. For elective surgery – that is operations that are planned rather than an emergency – people come into hospital reasonably fit, although they may still be debilitated by their condition. They may also have other conditions that need to be managed alongside, such as diabetes.

There are times, though, when a surgical ward can be more like A&E on a Saturday night, and none more so than a women's health or gynaecology ward. There are few emergencies quite like a vaginal haemorrhage or an ectopic pregnancy threatening to rupture to remind you that rapid life-saving action overthrows any lingering ritual and routine. An ectopic pregnancy occurs when a pregnancy develops outside the uterus, where there is not enough space for it to grow and so it can rupture causing a life threatening internal haemorrhage. Elizabeth says:

> One of our consultants did an emergency laparotomy in the scrub room. A woman arrived on the ward in a state of collapse with a ruptured ectopic. Her husband carried her through the ward doors and she was white as the proverbial sheet. All the theatres were occupied, so the consultant made the decision and off we went no pre op prep. The anaesthetist had worked in remote parts of Africa, he never batted an eye lid at difficult cases.

Happily, due to the swift action of nursing and medical staff, the woman lived.

Miscarriage is the most common complication of early pregnancy. One in four pregnancies are said to result in miscarriage and while this is always distressing for the parents, it is not something that is investigated, usually until a woman has experienced a third miscarriage.

In the past women were advised to rest if they thought they were miscarrying, although there is not much evidence that rest is effective, particularly in the early weeks. The advice, long ago, might also have included telling women to raise the foot of the bed at home (phone directories were good for this) to keep their blood pressure up.

Pain and vaginal bleeding are usually what herald a miscarriage and these need monitoring, particularly later in a pregnancy. Doreen was working nights on a gynae ward and a woman who was about twenty-three weeks pregnant came through the ward doors miscarrying. A full term pregnancy is forty weeks and twenty-three weeks is around the time when a pregnancy can be described as 'viable' – a baby might survive. Doreen and her colleagues leapt into action, delivered the woman and then ran with the baby boy to the special-care baby unit. He survived and is alive and well today.

Emergencies aside, patients are now in and out of hospital in no time. Even a woman having a hysterectomy may go home the same day if the surgery is done laparoscopically. In the 1980s, we used to admit those having such major gynaecological surgery two days before their operation for pubic shaves, for enemas, to have their bloods taken and even to have chest X-rays to be sure they were fit for anaesthetic. A generation before that it was usual for them to be admitted for a week before surgery and then be discharged to two weeks convalescence before going home. This absence from home did not always sit well with husbands.

Elizabeth recalls one young woman in her early 30s who came in for major gynaecological surgery:

> During the morning I received a telephone call from her husband, who was very cross. He said his wife had promised to ring when she came out of theatre and she hadn't. I explained she was recovering from anaesthesia. I asked if it was urgent, he said 'yes she was going to tell me how to use the washing machine'.

Women's health nursing is also, much like A&E, home to the curious and unusual. Mary Anne was approached by a young man who wanted her to ask the surgeon if he could please surgically cut his fiancée's hymen, as he didn't want to do it on the wedding night.

130

Requests to repair hymens were also reasonably common as women didn't want their husbands-to-be to know that they might have had sex with someone else. That sex is not the sole reason for a broken hymen, and that such surgery should even be requested, casts an almost medieval view of how women may still be regarded.

Foreign objects

Removal of foreign objects from different orifices is a frequent occurrence, although the variety of objects never ceases to amaze. A&E and women's health wards probably see most of these, which sometimes require anaesthesia and surgery to be removed, depending on the object. Sometimes they are referred to as Hasselhoff injuries – describing someone who presents with an injury for which there is a bizarre explanation. The source of this is an accident by the Baywatch actor David Hasselhoff (see medical slang glossary pp. 34).

Nikki reports patients presenting with £10 notes stuffed in their vaginas, frequent admissions of young girls with the tops of deodorant cans firmly stuck against their cervixes, as well as bathroom sponges and most weirdly of all on one occasion, fish hooks. Mary Anne says in A&E patients presented with all kinds: one with a key stuck in her vagina, another with a cricket ball in the rectum and still more astonishing, another with a gerbil in his back passage.

When I was training, there was a rumour that flew around the hospital that a woman had come into A&E with one or more snooker balls inside her vagina. The number seemed to increase with the telling of the story, and there were many lewd jokes about potting different colours. Far removed as I was from A&E, I hoped they might be considering that the woman was more than likely the victim of abuse and were offering her support, such that was available then.

One couple arrived on the ward on a stretcher locked in embrace. Nikki says: 'The woman had severe vaginismus during intercourse and the poor chap was stuck inside and in absolute agony. Red faces all round and an almost hysterical ambulance crew!'

A swift dose of a muscle relaxant and they were free of each other, with hopefully a fairly vague memory of what had just happened.

Chapter 12

Life and Death

'I have never felt so alone and cheated as at that moment.'

To experience not one but two deaths within your first few hours on a ward could put you off nursing altogether. Not so, Tom Bolger, former RCN head of education, whose first day as a nursing auxiliary brought more than a reasonable amount of death. Post A Levels and unsure what to do next, he signed up to be a nursing auxiliary at his local hospital. 'The hospital was a former workhouse. I was sent to the male surgical ward and assigned, together with a first year student nurse, to blanket bath a patient in a side room.'

No sooner had Tom embarked on his very first bed bath than the patient died. The student and Tom reported back to the charge nurse who, unperturbed, assigned them to blanket bath the patient in the other side room while he organised for the first patient to be washed and laid out. Tom and his new colleague started the second bed bath only for that patient to die too. Tom says: 'I don't ever remember being shocked about it.'

As Tom had discovered, there is an art to managing a ward so that the most ill are subject to the closest observation. On the long Nightingale wards, patients in side rooms in sight of the desk and those nearest the nurses' station tended to be the most ill. Patients just back from theatre were installed in a bed where the nurses could see them – although this is more difficult in these days of wards with bays. Patients picked up on what we thought was the discreet movement of the most ill up the ward so to be in view of the nurses' station.

I remember them anxiously asking if there had been a downturn in their condition as they found themselves moving closer to the nurses' desk. At that stage in my training, I didn't have a ready set of reassuring answers.

Margaret Lamb who worked at the RIE in the 1930s records in an RCN Oral History interview, that a certain Miss Renton did ward rounds after the night sister's report: medical one day, surgical the next. She only spoke to the patients in the surgical ward who were going to theatre. She was very religious and she just thought it was the right thing to do. However, the patients believed she only spoke to those she thought might not return from surgery and so hoped she wouldn't speak to them.

Superstition, along with rituals and myths, plays a big part in illness. It may be connected to people's cultural background or stigma around disease. Sometimes its origin is long forgotten. There are few nurses who will tolerate red and white flowers together in a vase. Some say there is a connection to the red and white of the War of the Roses, that they signify death and dying, blood and bandages.

In Sligo General Hospital, Berni remembers talk of the banshee: this Irish supernatural death messenger was traditionally seen or heard wailing or keening close to, or upon the time of, death, and was associated with families of Gaelic heritage, particularly those with surnames beginning with 'Mc' or 'Mac' or 'O' (such as McGrath or O'Brien). 'If the banshee was heard, you were supposed to rush around the ward and check all your patients to make sure they were still alive!'

There is also the sixth sense that animals have – a ginger cat that used to sit on the bed of hospice patients who were dying, while Eileen remembers Pussy Darling on the TB ward who would also curl up on the bed of a patient who was dying. Melissa's story, though, has to be the weirdest of all:

> I trained as a learning disability nurse in the 1980s. The hospital was in a rural location and there was an albino squirrel that was seen occasionally and was believed to predict death – which of course always came in threes.

This may be the same hospital in Canterbury where, rumour has it, students couldn't qualify as registered nurses unless they had seen the albino squirrel. How do you prove that you have seen it? No phones with cameras to hand in those days.

And there are rituals too, after death. When I trained, when someone died, they were always left for an hour after death and if possible, a window opened to allow their spirit or soul to leave. I think that hour is no longer respected as beds on busy wards are in such demand and nurses are required to move quickly to make it ready for a new admission. The experience in hospices is usually different, with more space and time given to friends and family of the deceased.

Until quite recently, care of the body after death was referred to as 'last offices', reminiscent of both the military and religious origins so familiar to nursing's history. Nurses have always been mindful to honour the spiritual or cultural wishes of the deceased person and their family, but the phrase 'care after death' is more usual now. Laying out a body is something every nurse has to do and as students we were anxious about this but discovered that it is often a peaceful and rewarding experience. It can also make you jump! I remember helping to turn a deceased patient in order to wash him and he exhaled noisily, startling myself and my colleague, making us laugh nervously as we remembered that when someone dies, they may well still have air in their lungs which is pushed out when they are moved.

Porters come to collect the body in a special trolley with a lid on it to take it to the mortuary – often referred to as Rose Cottage (not to be confused with Forces slang for the clap clinic). It was usually the student nurse's job to run round the ward and close the curtains around each patient's bed so they didn't witness the removal of the body. Yet they could all hear the ominous rattle of the metal trolley as it trundled down the ward.

Bodies were always removed feet first, this may have military origins but also may be simply practical, the upper part of a body is much heavier than the lower and so coffins are carried feet first. Superstition has it that the feet are leading the way to a new world and the body cannot look back at the one it is leaving.

Care and compassion

Although an inevitable part of life, especially in hospital, death and dying can still come as a shock not only to loved ones, but also to those caring for them. Almost everyone remembers their 'first death'. For me, it was less the death for which the ward sister had kindly prepared me and my co-student Mandy on our first placement, but more my shock when a friend of the deceased arrived the next day to visit him, unaware of his demise. As he asked for Mr Tring, I froze. I had no idea what to say. I was immensely grateful when another nurse stepped in and smoothly handled the situation.

She then spent time working alongside me as we stocked cupboards, assessing my level of distress, teasing out of me that my mother had just been diagnosed with lung cancer – the same illness that had carried off Mr Tring. That was when I appreciated what compassion was, although I couldn't name it at the time. To stay with someone in the moment can be so important. Although, I didn't find it quite so comforting when she said she and her mother were still grieving her father's death seventeen years down the line. That turned out to be another lesson.

Compassion for those who care has always tended to be in rather short supply in the caring professions and no one has ever really explained why. Is it about being professional, that we are merely the givers of care, that we don't have feelings? Social work has a system of supervision where someone can talk through their work issues and events with a more experienced colleague. This is recognised as an important aspect of the job, yet nothing similar has ever existed in nursing and medicine.

Fleur worked on oncology and found it both hugely rewarding and deeply distressing. For her it was all about total care of the patient, looking after them and their families and if a patient died, she would often go to the funeral. Her ward sister, seeing the effect this was having on Fleur advised her to: 'disinvest in patients and their relatives'.

Fleur says:

> She felt that if I was going to funerals I would burn out and it was better to invest in the task of nursing! I told her I'd rather give full care and burn out ... which I did in two years but I gave the most rewarding care.

My own experience of the death of a parent while a student closely mirrors that of Alison Collin who trained fifteen years before me at the same hospital. As Alison recounts in her book *Of Sluices and Sisters*, she was a second-year student reduced to tears while caring for a particular patient because he, like her father, had terminal cancer and her father had just been admitted to hospital. The ward sister, usually a formidable character who stood no nonsense from anyone, especially student nurses, immediately sent Alison off to matron's office to request compassionate leave. Unfortunately, as Alison says, compassion was only extended to patients, and matron, usually kindly disposed to students, informed her that the hospital was set up for the wellbeing of the patients and not the nurses and that Alison 'should tear myself away from my Mother's apron strings'.

Fortunately, the ward sister arranged for Alison to have an unscheduled weekend off and she was able to spend some time with her father – within the constraints of the strict visiting times of the day.

A couple of weeks later, she was summoned to matron's office and told her father had died. She was now allowed to go home. Alison says: 'I have never felt so alone and cheated as at that moment.'

Fifteen years later, I was three weeks into starting my nurse training when my mother was diagnosed with lung cancer. Six months later, I was a second warder working nights on a, forgive me, terminally dull observation ward. Tucked away discreetly above A&E, nothing much happened there – or if it did it usually concerned a medical student involved in some indiscretion who was quietly treated away from the prying eyes of the Nightingale wards. Student nurses could only guess – and frequently did – at the nature of these brief admissions.

While I was on nights my two brothers appeared on the ward to let me know that our mother had been admitted to a hospice and was now terminally ill.

Having never spoken of my mother's illness to anyone but my closest friends, I managed to convey this to the staff nurse, saying I needed to go home the next day. She was shocked and I assumed this was because it was a shocking thing to say, but it may have been the temerity of my saying I would not be back on duty for the foreseeable future. I told the night sister when she came by and she said: 'Well, we will have to see. You can't just leave your post.'

I don't remember her expressing any words of condolence. At the end of the shift I crossed the square to the nurses' home – a few metres away, bumping into two friends going on day shift. I let them know I was on my way home and why. I got changed and packed a few things, waited until 09.00 when the nursing offices opened. To this day I cannot remember who I spoke to, but she was very senior and very clear that nurses did not abandon their posts.

After the night sister's response, I had half expected this and I listened politely but was equally clear that I had informed the hospital of what

I was doing so I didn't think I was abandoning anything and I would go home. I think she weighed up just how vital I was as a second warder on a ward with five beds, only three of which were occupied, how likely it was that I would go anyway (very), and how this might reflect on the school of nursing, so after her homily she gave me permission to go. I stayed at home until after my mother's death and funeral some two weeks later before returning, quite raw, to complete my training.

Bereavement counselling was not a regular thing then, although it had been suggested by a nurse in the hospice and I had been non-plussed that any help should be offered to me or my family. Instead I struggled on while my friends did their best to be supportive in a situation that was entirely alien to all of us.

For Jacqui, it was those newly formed friendships that saw her through the trauma she experienced when her brother died just a week into our introductory block. Apart from attending his funeral she was not allowed compassionate leave. She was told she would have to drop out of the course and join another set later in the year. To her immense credit, she stayed on and went on to qualify. Having started to kindle early friendships – friendships that are still going strong today – it was important to stay among those who knew her story. There is nothing worse when you have been bereaved to have to explain your circumstances to new people time and again.

On the same ward as Mr Tring I remember a popular, ebullient patient called John who had taken a sudden turn for the worse after having been due for discharge. A couple of other nurses and I were sent off for our break only to discover on our return that pandemonium had broken out in those fifteen minutes, the crash team had been called and John had died as a result of septicaemia. The life and death nature of our jobs certainly hit home.

Another patient, Ron, who looked a bit like Sid James and was only slightly less saucy, was part of the fixtures and fittings. He knew the routine better than the nurses. He did the morning and evening drinks round – being careful to observe the fluid restrictions of various patients. I didn't know much about his condition until at handover I learnt that he was something of a walking timebomb. He had oesophageal varices – essentially varicose veins lining the tube to the stomach which could burst at any moment to spurt blood fountain like out of his throat. Oesophageal varices are associated with severe liver disease and in Ron's case, caused by a lifetime of too much alcohol.

Thereafter a Sengstaken tube was kept on Ron's locker. If the varices burst, this tube, which had little balloons one at the end and two near the top, was to be passed down Ron's nose or throat and the balloons inflated so they applied pressure to the veins to reduce bleeding. Red blankets were stored on the end of Ron's bed should they be needed. Originally a military concept, these were significant – if Ron were to haemorrhage, much of the horror would be absorbed in the red blankets. With all these preparations I found I was beginning to mentally disengage with Ron, to recognise that he was not likely to be going home and that his time might be very limited. Perhaps that's what we do as health professionals, disengage or maybe we don't engage in the first place so the patient fails to properly become a person to us?

It was still a shock to come onto shift one morning and receive the news that Ron's varices had indeed burst in the night and while the nurses and the crash team had done all they could, the haemorrhage was too immense to stem and he had died. The nurse giving handover was shocked at what she had witnessed and we all mourned the passing of a popular patient. But nothing more was said. No one spoke about that emotional loss. Maybe this is a very British stiff upper lip combined with the slightly detached professional persona.

Not for resus

The crash team is made up of doctors and nurses trained to help staff in medical emergencies including cardiac arrest. Often the least experienced person on the resus team is the youngest and fittest (a newly qualified F1) and they can find themselves first on the scene but terrified to suddenly be the decision maker. I know at least one F1 who did an extra lap of the corridors in his first month to make sure he didn't arrive first.

Etiquette, even for cardiac arrests, remained in place for too long. Martin witnessed a crash team in full swing at a cardiac arrest, with the ward sister, who was a petite woman, crouched on the bed in order to adequately perform cardiac massage. 'The man survived but I remember the sister subsequently received a dressing down for having knelt on the bed. Obviously to the powers-that-be, the dignity of nursing was more important than a man's life.'

The protocol for managing a cardiac arrest has changed markedly over the years as knowledge and technology have improved. When I was a student on my first two wards, I witnessed a patient arresting and did as we were taught then, thumped them on the chest and began cardiac massage, simultaneously pulling the alarm bell and calling for help.

On both occasions, the crash team arrived (not fast enough in my adrenaline-fuelled opinion) and a doctor decided the patient was 'not for resus'. Both were elderly, one a woman who had heart failure, whose family had not visited in weeks but suddenly turned up in angry numbers when she died, the other a Norwegian former sailor who didn't speak a word of English and had been living on the streets before he was brought in. An alcoholic, he had gone through severe DTs (delirium tremens) as he was weaned off alcohol, seeing monsters and spiders and shouting and thumping people who came close. And yet, I had grown fond of him and was shocked that his fate could be decided quite so casually (as I saw it). When a fellow student, who obviously hadn't grown fond of him, said it was about time, he was taking up a bed at great cost, I realised she was not the compassionate type.

These days, the decision over whether a patient should be resuscitated is, ideally, discussed with patient and family and recorded in the notes as DNACPR (do not attempt cardiopulmonary resuscitation) and all staff are informed.

The Big C

At one time, cancer was considered a death sentence. As such, doctors were often reluctant to tell patients their diagnosis. Thankfully this is quite rare these days because it creates an impossible secrecy, especially as patients will almost always want to talk, often in the middle of the night.

On my third ward – male surgical – Mr Jones had been a patient for some weeks. He was aware he had cancer but as far as he was concerned it was under control. He was not allowed to know his prognosis, which was poor. He was dying. I can't remember why he wasn't to know and can only imagine his family were trying to protect him. During my day shifts on the ward I felt enormously uncomfortable caring for him,

139

scared he was going to ask me how he was doing and being unsure just how I would respond. Inwardly I was furious that such crucial information was being kept from him.

I went onto a set of nights with Sarah, a staff nurse who was fun and capable and treated students as her equal. Mr Jones was deteriorating fast and one night I came back from my break and Sarah told me she had sat with Mr Jones and when he asked, she had told him he was dying. He said he was glad she had told him and he died some days later when I was off duty. When I returned to the ward, there was an envelope for me with £5 inside it and a note from Sarah saying Mr Jones had given us £10 to share as a thank you. I kept the note and £5 for many years before, I'm ashamed to say, I spent the money when I was especially broke. I still have the note.

In 1958, Joan remembers three patients coming in for major surgery for lung cancer. It was the routine that on the morning after surgery they had chest X-rays done on the ward so the results were available for the doctor's round at 10.00. It was Joan's job to prop up the patients so they could get the X-ray plates behind their backs. They were in a lot of pain and she would hold them upright while the X-ray was taken. While she wore a protective leaded apron, she did not have a thyroid shield to protect her.

In the same period, she nursed a man receiving treatment for cancer of the tongue. After surgery, he had sixteen radium needles placed in his tongue. He was nursed in the open ward and in what seems now to be totally inadequate protection. The nurses were advised to wear lead aprons and to sit behind him when feeding him so they were not directly exposed to the radium needles. It was an era when, perhaps unwittingly, the patient's comfort and dignity were placed above that of the nurse's safety.

Anyone working with radiation was required to wear a dosimeter – a little badge that recorded the amount of radiation to which they were exposed. Tests on Joan's dosimeter revealed that in two weeks she had exceeded the safe limits for X-rays and for radiation and was told not to go near X-rays again for the rest of her life except for herself, and only then in a life-saving capacity.

As a third-year student, I worked on a gynaecology ward, looking after a woman post-surgery for a pelvic cancer. She also had caesium rods. She used bed pans and the output was disposed of in special drums that would be taken away because of latent radioactivity. I was mortified when I tipped a bedpan full of radioactive urine down the usual sluice. I had visions of poisoning the whole of London; of fire officers in the 1980s equivalent of hazmat suits having to lift all the drain lids in the vicinity to try and catch the fateful urine. I had to confess! I tentatively approached the ward sister – she was young, I liked her and this was the first ward I had really enjoyed in three years of nursing – now it was all ruined.

As I approached, she turned to me and said with that ward sister sixth sense: 'you've thrown the urine down the sluice, haven't you?' As I nodded, she said 'don't worry about it', and resumed what she was doing. I was both relieved and dumbstruck – of all the things student nurses got into trouble for, this was surely genuinely serious and yet it was ignored. I suspect I was not the first to have made the mistake and quite possibly there was no protocol in place for dealing with such an error. The era of protocols was yet to come.

The unexpected

Traumatic events not preceded by months of illness are shocking for everyone, made worse when there is little time to prepare. This can happen in obstetrics when the expectation is of a happy event. As Mary Anne says:

> Obstetric theatres are the scene of some of the best and worst moments – the smiles and happy tears as a child is born and cries for the first time and then the utter devastation and sadness when a child is stillborn and there is silence. You look around the room and see everyone is taking a deep breath and holding back tears.

Being able to show a certain amount of emotion to relatives and, in this scenario, devastated parents, has to be good but has to be contained – it is the parents who are grieving, it is not for us to fill that space.

But as Adam Kay describes with crystal clarity in *This is Going to Hurt*, there is little or no formal assistance or supervision for the individuals in the healthcare team. What help there is comes from colleagues who may or may not have the emotional capacity to be there for you. To have a supportive home life is often all that can get you through, but even then it can be difficult to share with those who can't really comprehend the experience.

While good nursing care is about managing and monitoring your patients, being aware of their condition, it also involves the ability to deal with virtually any situation, calmly and constructively. Very often, such situations involve a sudden death.

It was early morning, about an hour before the end of shift at St Thomas's A&E where Mary Anne was a staff nurse, when a call came through to say a man on a coach had collapsed and the driver had been advised to go to the nearest A&E. When it arrived, the coach was too big to drive up the ramp to the entrance so had to park on London's embankment.

The coach was full of pensioners on their way to the airport for a winter holiday in Spain. Sid and his wife, Ava, had got on the coach at Aldwych (a few miles up the road) and after reaching up to put some bags in the overhead rack, Sid collapsed into his seat. Ava said she had been nagging him to hurry up and not keep people waiting. Then she couldn't wake him.

Mary Anne was first on the coach because the house officer, recognising her consummate ability to manage such a difficult situation, suggested that the sight of a uniform would calm people. It was obvious that Sid was dead. All the passengers were asked to disembark while she and the house officer worked out how to transfer Sid off the bus in a reasonably dignified manner. The staff in A&E provided tea for all forty passengers as they streamed, disorientated, into the department.

There was some confusion as to who was allowed to carry the body from the coach. Sid was not an inpatient in the hospital so it was not the hospital porters' job. The paramedics had not been called so it was not their job, so the morgue staff said they would do it – but they had to do it at the morgue, not out on the street. The driver had to inch the coach down the steep narrow slip road to the morgue so Sid could be removed as discreetly as possible.

It then parked back on the embankment, now in the middle of London's rush hour, ready for the passengers to board again, minus Sid and Ava. Their luggage had to be extracted from the coach. Mary Anne says: 'Someone passing took a photo and it appeared in one of the London evening papers with us with luggage hooks in hand delving into the depths of the coach, frilly hats and all.'

Bibliography

Books

Ashdown M.A., *A Complete System of Nursing*, JM Dent & Sons Ltd.

Baly M.E., *Nursing and Social Change,* 3rd edition, Routledge, London and New York.

Barton D., *The New Nightingale Chronicles* (newnightingalechronicles. blogspot.com).

Bellman L., Boase S., Rogers S., and Stuchfield B., *Nursing Through the Years: Care and Compassion at the Royal London Hospital*, Pen & Sword Books, Barnsley, 2018.

Collin A., *Of Sluices & Sisters,* Writersworld Woodstock, Oxford, 2009.

Funnell E., *Aids to Hygiene for Nurses,* Third ed. Balliere, Tindall and Cox, London, 1948.

Groves, Brickdale & Nixon, *Text Book for Nurses: Anatomy, Physiology, Surgery and Medicine,* sixth ed. Oxford University Press, London, 1940.

Hainsworth M., (ed.), *Modern Professional Nursing,* Volumes II, III and IV, Second ed. Caxton Publishing Co. Ltd, London, 1949.

Houghton M., *Aids to Theatre Technique*, Second ed. Balliere, Tindall and Cox, London, 1946.

Justham D., '"Those maggots – they did a wonderful job": The nurses' role in wound management in civilian hospitals during the Second World War', in Jane Brooks and Christine E. Hallett (eds), *One Hundred Years of Wartime Nursing Practices, 1854–1954*, Manchester University Press, 2015.

Kalisch P., & Kalisch B., *The Advance of American Nursing*, 3rd ed. J.B. Lipincott Company, Philadelphia, 1995.

Kay A., *This is Going to Hurt: Secret Diaries of a Junior Doctor*, Picador, 2017.

Menzies Lyth I., Social Systems as a Defence against Anxiety; An empirical study of the nursing service of a general hospital (A shortened version of the original Human Relations, 13:95-121, 1960) accessed September 2018.

Mortimer B., in association with the Royal College of Nursing, *Sisters Memories from the Courageous Nurses of World War Two*, Hutchinson, London, 2012.

Squibbs A., *Materia Medica For Nurses*, second edition Balliere, Tindall & Cox.

Walsh M., Ford P., *Nursing Rituals: Research and Rational Actions,* Butterworth Heinemann, 1989.

Watson J., *Aids to Fevers for Nurses,* Second ed. Balliere, Tindall and Cox, London, 1946.

Journals and papers

Al-Allak A., Sarasin S., Key S., Morris-Stiff G., (2008) 'Wedding Rings are not a Significant Source of Bacterial Contamination Following Surgical Scrubbing' 2008 Mar; 90(2): 133–135 (accessed Jan 18 2019)

Barberis, et al (2017) 'The history of tuberculosis: from the first historical records to the isolation of Koch's bacillus', *Journal of Preventive Medicine and Hygiene*; 58(1): E9–E12.

Biley F. and Wright S., (1997) 'Towards a defence of nursing routine and ritual', *Journal of Clinical Nursing,* Vol 6 pp115-119.

Catanzaro A.M., (2002) 'Beyond the Misapprehension of Nursing Rituals', Nursing Forum, Vol 37. No. 2 April–June.

Clark D., (2014) 'The Brompton Cocktail: 19th century origins to 20th century demise' http://endoflifestudies.academicblogs.co.uk/thebrompton-cocktail-19th-century-origins-to-20th-century-demise/ accessed May 2017

Evans A.M., Pereira D.A., Parker J.Mn., (2008) 'Discourses of anxiety in nursing practice: a psychoanalytic case study of the change-of-shift handover ritual', *Nursing Inquiry*.15, 1, 40-48.

Fretwell, (1982) *Ward Teaching and Learning*, RCN, London.

Garrett, B., Singiser, D., and Banks, S., (1992) 'Back injuries among nursing personnel: the relationship of personal characteristics, risk factors, and nursing practices.' AAOHN Journal, 40:11, pp. 510–516.

Justham D., (2014) 'A Study of Nursing Practices Used in the Management of Infection in Hospitals, 1929–1948'. PhD thesis, University of Manchester. This online PDF resource can be found at https://www.library.manchester.ac.uk/Chapter 7 explores wound care.

Katz P., (1981) 'Ritual in the operating room'. Ethnology 20, 335–350 (theatres).

Lathan R., (2010) Caroline Hampton Halsted: the first to use rubber gloves in the operating room (Bayl Univ Med Cent) 2010 Oct; 23(4): 389–392. PMCID: PMC2943454 (accessed 10 November, 2018).

Mann, E., and Redwood, S., (2000) 'Improving Pain Management: Breaking Down the Invisible Barrier', *British Journal of Nursing*, Vol 9, no 19, pp 2067–2072.

Oral histories. With thanks to the RCN for access to their oral history interviews. Repository code: GB1199. The following oral histories were used in part:

GB1199 T/16 Alice Kemp (nee Bryan)

GB1199 T/17 Margaret Lamb

GB1199 T/258 Kathleen Hutchison,

GB1199 T/139 Evelyn Davies,

GB1199 T/34 Winifred Hector

GB1199 T/428 Mary Brown (nee Dawson)

Pearson A., Baker H., Walsh K., and Fitzgerald M., (2001) 'Contemporary Nurses' Uniforms – History and Traditions', *Journal of Nursing Management.*

Philpin S., (2002) 'Rituals and nursing: a critical commentary', *Journal of Advanced Nursing* 38(2), 144–151.

Philpin S., (2006) 'Information Transmission in ITU nurses', British Association of Critical Care Nurses.

Scovell S., (2010) 'Role of the Nurse-to-Nurse Handover in Patient Care', *Nursing Standard*. 24, 20, 35–39.

Sleep J., Grant A., (1988) 'Effects of Salt and Savlon Bath Concentrate Post-Partum', *Nursing Times,* May 25–31:84(21):55–7.

The Londonist (2016) 'Who Exactly Are The Ghosts of London?' https://londonist.com/2016/10/who-exactly-are-the-ghosts-of-london

Thurgood, G., 'A History of Nursing in Halifax and Huddersfield 1870–1960', (thesis submitted for PhD, University of Huddersfield, 2008) This version is available at http://eprints.hud.ac.uk/id/eprint/8353/

Thurgood, Graham (2005) 'Defining Moments in Medical History – Nurses' Narratives of their Everyday Experiences of a Key 20th Century Historical Event – the First Use of Antibiotics' In: *Narrative, Memory & Everyday Life,* University of Huddersfield, Huddersfield, pp. 231–242. This version is available at http://eprints.hud.ac.uk/4959/

Tucker A., Fox P., (2014) 'Evaluating Nursing Handover: The REED Model', *Nursing Standard*. 28, 20, 44–48.

Blogs

Al-Rais, A.S., (2017) How to avoid handover hostility BMJ (accessed 27 August 2018) https://blogs.bmj.com/bmj/2017/01/13/andrew-s-alrais-how-to-avoid-handover-hostility/

Websites

The 6Cs NHS England https://www.england.nhs.uk/leadingchange/about/the-6cs/ (accessed 1 May 2019)

Events and meetings

Nurses' Tales (2018) personal stories from nurses over the seventy years of the NHS; Accounts from Ann Keen, Christine Hancock, Jan Williams.

St Bartholomew's League of Nurses October 2017 and 2018. Anecdotes from League nurses including Natalie Doyle.

Index